TESTIMONIALS

TO WHOM IT MAY CONCERN

RE: Dr. Rao Konduru's Publications:
    Reversing Obesity
    Reversing Sleep Apnea
    Reversing Insomnia

Dr. Rao Konduru, PhD is a patient of mine who has suffered from chronic diabetes for most of his life. He also suffered from uncontrollable obesity, sleep apnea and chronic insomnia for the past 3 to 4 years. He has managed to reverse all of these conditions by taking non-pharmacological and science-based natural measures with great success. He has created 3 how-to user guides/books with regard to how he achieved this, and I recommend these books for anyone suffering from these conditions.

Sincerely,
Dr. Ali Ghahary, MD
Brentwood Medical Clinic
Burnaby, British Columbia, Canada

At first we read "Reversing Obesity" another book by Dr. RK, and we found it better than the best books in the weight-loss industry. His recipe for the pre-workout meal "Egg White Omelet" is a major highlight. Anyone can lose weight by eating whole foods and by following the simple instructions for rapid weight loss method illustrated by Dr. RK.

After that we read his second book "Reversing Sleep Apnea" and we were blown away by its extremely impressive contents. Dr. RK convinces you beyond a shadow of a doubt that obstructive sleep apnea can be reversed simply and easily by losing weight. He has covered all the important therapies that a sleep apnea patient would ever need.

Then we read his third book "Reversing Insomnia" and his writing keeps getting more and more interesting. Dr. RK describes exactly where the planet Earth is located in our universe, and how it creates the daytime and nighttime by rotating on its own axis and by revolving around the sun. He divides the 24-hour master biological clock into two parts, one for the daytime and the other for the nighttime, and instructs the insomniacs what to do exactly as the day progresses and as the night progresses. By simply following his instructions, naturally, and without ever using sleeping pills, anyone can reset his/her master biological clock, and sleep like a baby within a few days. What a wonderful book!
 - Prime Publishing Co.
New Westminster, British Columbia, Canada

This book "Reversing Insomnia" is the simplest, and perhaps the safest way to cure chronic insomnia. Dr. RK has done all the spadework and leaves the rest of us to reap the benefits. All one has to do is read and follow the simple do-it-yourself instructions.

Hats off to Dr. RK and his impressive research. He figured how the master biological clock embedded in the brain works, and came up with an effortless and natural method to permanently cure chronic insomnia. He applied and tested his discovery on himself. It took him just 3 days to reverse his chronic insomnia after suffering from it for over 3 years.

After reading the entire book, I wholeheartedly believe it is the best cure for the sleep disorder. One, because it hardly takes time to cure the insomnia; two, because it has no side effects; and three, because sleeping pills are a complete waste of money.

It really works. So, just give it a try!

- Ms. Muriel D'Souza, Advertising Copywriter, Vancouver, British Columbia, Canada

----

++

REVIEWS

Please do not ignore reviews. Please read all reviews thoroughly.
You can learn a lot by reading through the reviews below:

++

Jade
5.0 out of 5 stars The Natural and Effortless Insomnia Treatment That Works!
Reviewed in the United States on February 5, 2021
Verified Purchase

Until the electricity was discovered and distributed for modern living, and before the houses, workplaces and streets were illuminated by electricity, our ancestors used to work hard under the Sunlight during the day, and used to sleep in pitch-black dark houses during the night. Our ancestors did not suffer from chronic insomnia like we do now by living under bright and powerful electric lamps in houses, workplaces and on streets. This is the major cause of current-day chronic insomnia.

This book "Reversing Insomnia" teaches that by living under the Sunlight or bright lights during the day (for 12 hours), and by living strictly in the pitch-black darkroom during the night without ever exposing to
bright lights (for another 12 hours) at least for a few days, it is possible to reset the Master Biological Clock, and to reverse chronic insomnia. This is the fundamental principle based on which the method of reversing chronic insomnia has been derived and outlined in this book.

All we need do is reset "the Master Biological Clock" by doing some simple exercises nicely outlined in this book in a simple language in order to reverse chronic insomnia.
If you read, understand and follow carefully all 24 instructions outlined in the Main Article of this book in Chapter 1, you can reverse chronic insomnia in 3 days to 3 weeks, depending on how seriously and sincerely you implement this method without breaking the rules.

I reversed it in 3 days. It is the one 100% natural method. All those prescription sleeping pills and OTC sleep aids are a mere waste of money, unnecessary and they further ruin your health. Believe it or not, this natural method works but you must try it seriously and sincerely by exercising self-discipline at least for a few days! All sleep clinics should adopt this natural method. All insomniacs must be free from insomnia by using this book.

++

Wang Inhee
5.0 out of 5 stars Nice!
Reviewed in the United States on November 8, 2019   Format: Kindle Edition
I would highly recommend everyone to read this book. This book gave me a lot of information. This book is awesome to read and I think this book is the best book of this topic, and I really appreciate this book.

++

++

Jailyn *5.0 out of 5 stars* Helpful Steps to Treat Insomnia!
Reviewed in the United States on November 4, 2020 Verified Purchase

Computers, laptops, iPads, iPhones, tablets, cell phones, many other gadgets, and bright light bulbs at home, workplace, and outdoors, they all attack our eyes with "artificial bright light late at night," tricking our body's master biological clock into living at a perpetual high noon (12 o'clock in the daytime), mimicking the sunlight. The brain therefore enters into a state of confusion, and becomes unable to recognize that it is the night time, and does not secrete the natural melatonin as usually from the pineal gland (which is a fluid-filled space located on the back of the brain), thereby developing insomnia or chronic insomnia. Natural production of melatonin from the pineal gland of your brain is essential to fall asleep and to maintain deep sleep at night, especially late at night.

"Reversing Insomnia: The Instant Guide to Sleeping Like A Baby Tonight" provides us very simple "Do-It-Yourself Instructions" on how to reset the master biological clock and how to reverse chronic insomnia through simple exercises so that the melatonin production from pineal gland becomes normalized. Just follow the 24 simple instructions outlined in this course in the first chapter, and you will be able to reset master biological clock, and reverse chronic insomnia. It is possible to reverse it in 3 days if you try it seriously. Right from the first night, when you start living alone in a pitch-black room, you will start yawning excessively with an instant feeling of sleeping. That means you are on your way to reversing chronic insomnia.

Reversing Insomnia book has taught me so many wonderful things and deeds to naturally treat and reverse my chronic insomnia, and so I adore this book!
++

rohit joshi *5.0 out of 5 stars* Real Insomnia Cure Is At Your Fingertips!
Reviewed in India on March 4, 2020 Verified Purchase

I have been living with insomnia for a long time, and those sleeping pills are not at all helping me. My body created resistance to sleeping pills, and they stopped working. I may have to increase the dosage of sleeping pills in order to make them work, but it would be dangerous to do so, as this book suggests.

This effortless sleep method and natural self-treatment explained nicely in the book "Reversing Insomnia" is very easy to practice, and it works like a miracle right from the first day. All I needed was Chapter 1 to reverse my insomnia. I read Chapter 1, I did not even read the whole book, and I started seeing results immediately.

The weather where I live is very hot, and I can easily expose to sunshine during the day as explained in this book, which has helped boost my sleep at night. I have maintained darkness at my home easily by turning off all the lights. I just used my torch light to move within my small house. Voila, everything worked like a miracle as explained in this book when I started living in pitch-black room. I started yawning and was tempted to go to bed early. I slept on my side as this book suggests, and woke up in the morning fully refreshed.

I am so grateful for all those 24 instructions detailed in Chapter 1, and very useful information outlined in the other chapters. Every chapter has interesting information. All that information about caffeine control in Chapter 7 will also be very useful to me. I genuinely recommend this book to whoever suffers from chronic insomnia. This natural method works, just try it out!
++

+++

Anna Zoe
4.0 out of 5 stars Appreciating content
Reviewed in the United States on November 6, 2019
Format: Kindle Edition

I was recommended this book by a sleep specialist. It is helping me a lot. I can't thank the authors enough for the wonderful work they did writing it. They created a clear path to help with sleep issues; easy to follow directions, a bit of tough love and wonderful suggestions that make sense. Each step is explained well.

+++

Anamaría Aguirre Chourio
5.0 out of 5 stars No-Nonsense Insomnia Treatment!
Reviewed in the United States on March 9, 2020
Verified Purchase

After reading the very impressive books "(i) Drinking Water Guide, (ii) Permanent Diabetes Control, (iii) The Secret to Controlling Type 2 Diabetes" authored by Dr. RK, I decided to purchase and read his "Reversing Insomnia" book as well.

PERFECTLY NATURAL SELF-TREATMENT: This book's message is that we should live under sunlight or bright lights during the day, and in the dark during the night at least for a few days to reverse insomnia. In addition, by controlling the number of cups of coffee consumption, we can control the chronic sleeplessness. I must minimize the number of cups of coffee I consume daily or the amount of caffeine consumption per day by trial and error. Whatever amount of coffee I decided to consume must be consumed before noon (No coffee consumption in the afternoon).

Living in the pitch-black darkness during the night after 7 pm is of utmost importance during the insomnia treatment until the chronic insomnia is completely reversed and until you are free. Going out and exposing to street bright lights is prohibited so stay home all the night when on this insomnia treatment. There are many other instructions to be followed (there are 24 instructions all together) rigorously to reset the Master Biological Clock located in the brain in order to achieve successful results.

REVERSING INSOMNIA book contains a natural insomnia self-treatment method, which is very practical and it works. All naturopathic doctors will be elated to read this book, and to know about this perfectly natural and no-nonsense self-treatment. This method should be adopted by all insomniacs. This method worked for me, as I easily reversed my sleeplessness in a few days without spending a dime. I am sure it will work for anybody as long as the person follows all 24 Do-It-Yourself instructions at least for a few days.

+++

++

Deanna Maio
5.0 out of 5 stars Awesome Insomnia Course That Is Fully Natural!
Reviewed in the United States on August 30, 2020
Verified Purchase

This insomnia course made perfect sense to me as I was able to reverse my chronic insomnia in a few days by reading through chapter 1.

Common sense tells us that we must perfectly be awake during the day, and perfectly be asleep during the night. That was the reason why our planet Earth by rotating on its own axis every day (24 hours) and by revolving around the Sun in 365 days (1 year) creates day and night (12 hours for the day and 12 hours for the night).

During the day we are supposed to be perfectly awake and work hard under the sunlight, and during the night we are supposed to rest and sleep under the moonlight in the dark. The Master Biological Clock located in our brains is designed in such a way that it works perfectly well when we live under the Sun or bright lights during the day, and rest and sleep during the night by staying in the dark.

But the modern technology created electricity and everything changed. People started abusing the technological advancements by spending a lot of time sitting under artificial bright light. This kind of activity tricks your body's biological clock into living a perpetual noon, mimicking the bright sunlight. Therefore the pineal gland located in your brain fails to secrete natural melatonin. As a result, a person develops circadian rhythm disorder. This is the reason why some people fall asleep during the day and stay awake in the night, and feel the symptoms of underlying sleep disorder called "Chronic Insomnia".

++

Steve_M
5.0 out of 5 stars A Must-Read Book for All Insomniacs!
Reviewed in the United States on June 15, 2021
Verified Purchase

It is the safest way to cure chronic insomnia from its root causes. The author of this book has done an impressive research and, all the spadework, and leaves the rest of us to reap the benefits. All you need do is read and follow the simple do-it-yourself instructions.

This book explains how the master biological clock embedded in the brain works, and the author came up with an effortless and natural method to permanently cure chronic insomnia. He applied and tested his discovery on himself. It took him just 3 days to reverse his chronic insomnia after suffering from it for over 3 years.

After reading the entire book, I practiced it on myself, and it works exactly as it says. I wholeheartedly believe that it is the best cure for the chronic insomnia developed due to sleep disorder. You don't need to go to a sleep specialist who would prescribe you an anxiety pill. This natural method has no side effects, and remember the sleeping pills and anxiety pills are completely waste of money and worthless. You must read this book if you suffer from chronic insomnia.

++

++

Jack mckeever
5.0 out of 5 stars   Middle-of-the-Night Insomnia Cure Outlined!
Reviewed in the United Kingdom on March 2, 2020
Verified Purchase

I was indeed fascinated by this book's extraordinary contents and teachings on reversing insomnia. We often worry about lying awake in the middle of the night - but it could be good for you, some sleep specialists and researchers say. A growing body of evidence from both science and history suggests that the eight-hour continuous sleep may be unnatural.

Dr. THOMAS WEHR's RESEARCH ON SEGMENTED SLEEP: In the early 1990s, psychiatrist Dr. Thomas Wehr conducted an experiment in which a group of people were plunged into darkness for 14 hours every day for a month. It took some time for their sleep to regulate but by the fourth week the subjects had settled into a very distinct sleeping pattern. They slept first for four hours, then woke for one or two hours before falling into a second four-hour sleep. Though sleep scientists were impressed by the study, among the general public the idea that we must sleep for eight consecutive hours still persists.

This book suggests that "Segmented Sleep" should not be practiced intentionally. But if your sleep is divided into several segments during the night, stay peacefully in a relaxed mood as if everything was normal without panicking. Chapter 4 is dedicated for this kind of very interesting research-based topic. Living alone in the DARK ROOM (PITCH-BLACK ROOM) during the nighttime, without any kind of light (a battery-powered lamp can be used during walking only), would significantly help improve your sleep and combat chronic insomnia. The spontaneous melatonin production by the pineal gland located in your brain is the key to attaining a good night's sleep (Do not take artificial melatonin pills).

MY RECOMMENDATION: If you are suffering from middle-of-the night insomnia, refer to the main article of this course and read the Instruction # 24 of Chapter 1 "How to treat Middle-of-the-Night Insomnia," and follow the treatment method explained there step-by-step.

++

Daniele D'Alessio
5.0 out of 5 stars INSOMNIA TREATMENT IS EXPLAINED IN ONE PAGE!
Reviewed in the United Kingdom on August 24, 2020
Verified Purchase

CHRONIC INSOMNIA NATURAL TREATMENT IS SUMMARIZED IN ONE PAGE ONLY (Page 10 of the Book). You don't need to read the whole book to understand how to reverse chronic insomnia. By following these simple instructions provided in one page only, you can easily reverse your insomnia.

I had amazing experience with this book. It is completely a natural method, as we don't need to take any kind sleeping pills or OTC (over-the-counter) sleep remedies or sleep aids. In fact this book warns that we must not use sleep aids or prescription sleeping pills, and should reverse chronic insomnia naturally by understanding how the mater biological clock works, and by learning how to reset the Master Biological Clock. If you can reset the Master Biological Clock, you will be free from insomnia.

A person suffering from chronic insomnia can reset his/her Master Biological Clock in one day, in a few days, in a week, or in a month depending on how chronic the developed insomnia is, and how committed a person is to implement the treatment procedure. Each person is different so each person needs unique period of recovery time to re-programs his/her Master Biological Clock. We need to try it seriously by focusing on the natural method, without breaking any rule, and fully committed. High-self discipline and high willpower are required during this treatment period to achieve successful results (at least during the first week). If you understand all instructions and learn how to implement all instructions in this natural treatment, you will be free of insomnia, and start sleeping like a baby tonight. You should try it out! Please don't live like an insomniac by being addicted to sleeping pills!

+++

Chandan
5.0 out of 5 stars Chronic Insomnia Recovery Guide!
Reviewed in India on January 25, 2021
Verified Purchase

This book represents the "Chronic Insomnia Recovery Guide!" Reversing Insomnia book teaches how the Mater Biological Clock located in the brain works, and how the melatonin is naturally secreted from the pineal gland located in the brain. If we can reset the Master Biological Clock, the chronic insomnia can be reversed, and we can sleep like a baby afterwards. The author provides 24 easy-to-follow instructions to reset the Master Biological Clock.

DURING THE DAY: We essentially live under the Sunlight or under bright lights.
DURING THE NIGHT: We essentially live in the pitch-black darkness (be very strict!).

All those insomnia clinics must be wasting their time and money to treat chronic insomnia. All they need is this guide. I recommend this fantastic guide to all insomnia clinics, psychiatrists and all naturopathic doctors who should read this book, understand it thoroughly, and should prescribe this natural method to their insomnia patients, and should ask them to practice this natural treatment to become free from insomnia without ever taking any sleeping pills.

However you must read and understand all 24 instructions explained in Chapter 1 of this book, and put those instructions into practice to become free from chronic insomnia. If practiced seriously and sincerely, this natural method would work for anybody.

+++
Read more reviews on Amazon.com.
Search the book "Reversing Insomnia: The Instant Guide to Sleeping Like a Baby Tonight."

+++

++

Wellness Books
5.0 out of 5 stars   Effortless Sleep Method & Natural Insomnia Cure!
Reviewed in Canada on March 4, 2020
Verified Purchase

I recommend this "REVERSING INSOMNIA" book to all people suffering from sleeplessness or chronic insomnia.

Dr. RK'S BOOKS ARE ALL MUST-READ HEALTH BOOKS: I have read his intriguing book "Drinking Water Guide". His book "Permanent Diabetes Control" is wonderful. All his health books are extremely impressive, extremely interesting, extremely useful, and directly applicable to current-day health problems that many people face today. I recommend that both medical doctors and naturopathic doctors should read these books, and benefit from the contents. All his books are science-based and practical guides. His extensive scientific research experience is clearly visible in these books.

He teaches everything so nicely step-by-step by dividing the book's contents into many headings, sub-headings and paragraphs so that a layperson can easily understand his teachings. He always convinces the reader with logic by making simple calculations that make sense. All his teachings are science-based with simple mathematics and attractive tables, showing the innovative experiments he conducted at the comfort of his home on his own body, resolving his own complex health issues with natural methods, without ever using traditional prescription drugs being prescribed by doctors. This book is no different.

I have read and enjoyed his three well-written and well-organized books "Reversing Obesity, Reversing Sleep Apnea, and Reversing Insomnia." These books are extremely useful to medical community. All contents are directly applicable to my own health problems I have been facing for years, and extremely useful. I am now using his books and am sure these books will help me controlling my weight gain, my mild sleep apnea and help cure my insomnia (sleeplessness) as well. I offer my hearty congratulations to the author Dr. RK.

++

Antonie Brown
5.0 out of 5 stars   Recommended
Reviewed in the United States on November 6, 2019
Format: Kindle Edition
I purchased this book for my female friend who has trouble getting a full nights sleep. She often wakes up in the middle of the night and stays awake for hours. She read a lot of books on the subject. And she thought that this book provided the best information. The book is easy to read.

++

++

Poonam
5.0 out of 5 stars   Say Good Bye to Those Addictive Sleeping Pills!
Reviewed in India on January 27, 2021
Verified Purchase

Mark my words: this very easy natural method illustrated in this book in 24 steps works perfectly. I tried it and it worked for me absolutely one hundred percent to my fullest satisfaction, and I am certain that it would work for anybody suffering from chronic insomnia. All a person should do is read this book sincerely and seriously, and follow all instructions carefully, and then live in the darkness without exposing to bright lights during night after 7 pm. This method definitely works. Say good bye to sleeping pills. It costs only a tiny fraction of a sleeping pills prescription to purchase this book.

Visiting those sleep specialists, taking those expensive sleeping pills, or taking that artificial melatonin to promote sleep is unnecessary and naive. All a chronic insomnia patient needs is this book to reverse your chronic insomnia. I fully agree with the subtitle of this book "Instant Guide to Sleeping Like A Baby Tonight." I salute the author for compiling and putting together those 24 very interesting instructions that help relieve chronic insomnia, and for writing this concise book to help insomniacs. Every insomniac must read this book, reverse insomnia in a few days, and start sleeping like a baby thereafter. I wish all insomniacs "All the Best!"

++

Reema
5.0 out of 5 stars This Method Cures Chronic Insomnia from Its Root Causes!
Reviewed in India on March 11, 2021
Verified Purchase

This is an incredibly easy and miraculously natural method to reverse chronic insomnia from its root causes. That is how the chronic insomnia must be treated (it must be reversed from its root causes exactly as this book teaches). A friend of mine suggested me this book, and I was eager to know about this natural method as I have been wasting a lot of time and money to treat my chronic insomnia by visiting sleep specialists. Based on my opinion and my past experience, all kinds of sleeping pills must be banned and removed from the pharmacies. This natural method works exactly as described in this book without any help from sleeping pills. I reversed my chronic insomnia in a few days.

ALL YOU GOT TO DO IS: Reset your master biological clock if you suffer from chronic insomnia. You can do it in one day, one week, or in one month. Right on the first night when you start treating the circadian rhythm disorder following carefully the instructions outlined in this course by turning off the lights in the evening and by living in the dark, you would notice yourself yawning excessively and you will feel like sleeping. After practicing it for a few days seriously, you will start sleeping like a baby every night. Don't take my word for it and check it out with your own experience. You will be amazed!

++

Reversing Insomnia

The Instant Guide To Sleeping Like A Baby Tonight

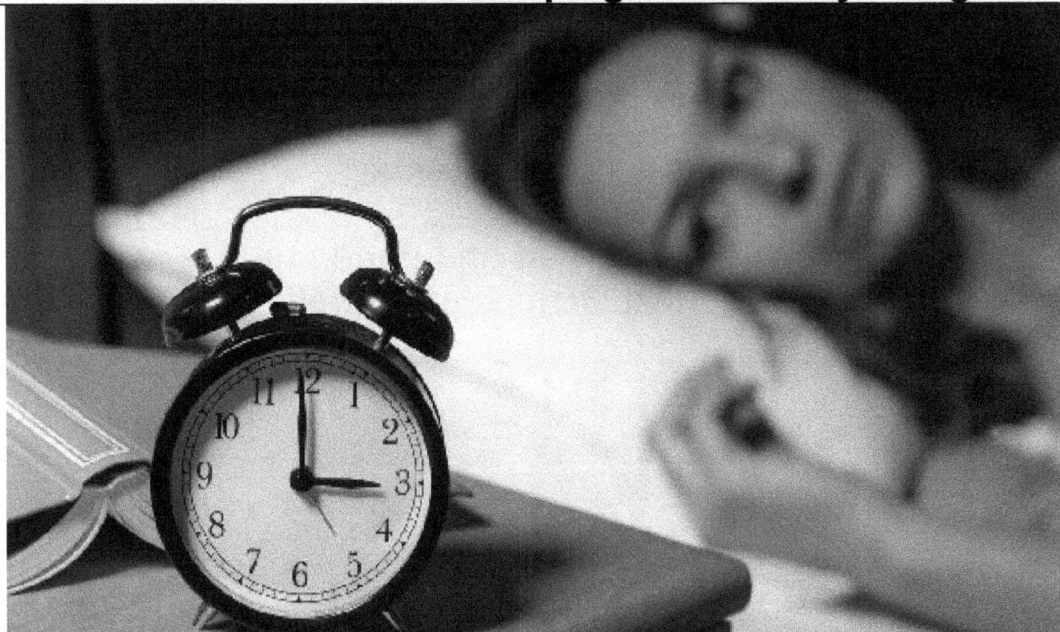

THIS EFFORTLESS SLEEP METHOD AND NATURAL SELF-TREATMENT IS THE ANSWER
To Cure Chronic Insomnia By Offsetting the Root Causes
Without Ever Using Any Sleeping Pills!

LEARN WHAT TO DO EXACTLY

DURING THE DAY	DURING THE NIGHT
• As the Day Begins	• As the Night Begins
• As the Day Progresses	• As the Night Progresses
• As the Day Ends	• As the Night Ends

EASY-TO-FOLLOW & DO-IT-YOURSELF INSTRUCTIONS
To Cure Chronic Insomnia Overnight!
This Guide Will Make You A Self-Taught Insomnia Guru!

Author: Rao Konduru, PhD

IMPORTANT NOTE

CHRONIC INSOMNIA TREATMENT IS SUMMARIZED IN ONE PAGE,
PLEASE REFER TO PAGE 10 IN THE PAPERBACK.

BY FOLLOWING THESE SIMPLE INSTRUCTIONS PROVIDED
IN ONE PAGE ONLY (You don't have to read the whole book),
YOU CAN EASILY REVERSE CHRONIC INSOMNIA IN 3 DAYS.
IT IS ABSOLUTELY POSSIBLE!

However please read and understand
the 24 detailed instructions of the full course.

FOREWORD

The Master Biological Clock located in the brain of every human being coordinates all the body clocks so that they are in synch. Each body clock has its own function. The Mast er Biological clock is made up of a group of about 20,000 nerve cells in the brain called Suprachiasmatic Nucleus (SCN), and is located in the hypothalamus, just above the optic nerve, and its major function is to control circadian rhythms.

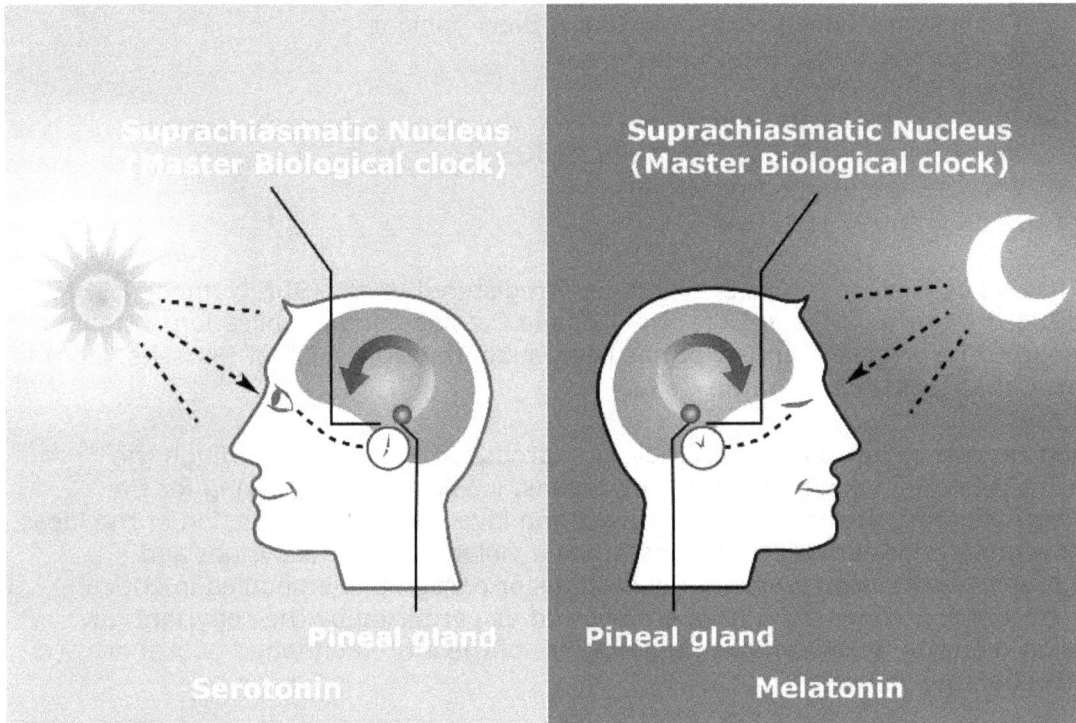

Figure 1 Sunshine promotes serotonin and moonlight promotes melatonin.

Sunlight, by passing through the retinas of our eyes, enters the hypothalamus and tells the Master Biological Clock the time of the day. The intensity of the sunlight is highly responsible for the production of serotonin that induces the feeling of joy. Moonlight and the intensity of darkness signal the Master Biological Clock, and in turn the pineal gland, that it is nighttime and it is the time to secrete melatonin. The melatonin production tells your body that it is time to sleep. Melatonin does not induce sleep, but it is up to the individual to understand the body's language (it is time to sleep), and to stay in a quiet and calm darkroom, to relax by suppressing all thoughts of the mind, and to go to bed in an attempt to sleep.

By living under sunlight or bright lights during the day, and by living strictly in the dark during the night, without exposure to bright lights, it is possible to reverse chronic insomnia. This is the fundamental principle based on which the method of reversing chronic insomnia has been derived and outlined in this book.

It is not that difficult to treat chronic insomnia. You absolutely do not need sleeping pills. If you read, understand and follow carefully all 24 instructions outlined in the Main Article of this book, you can reverse chronic insomnia in 3 days to 1 week (maximum 2 weeks). The reversal of insomnia begins right on the first night. You will feel it, yawning excessively as the night progresses. Believe it or not, Dr. RK reversed his chronic insomnia in 3 days after suffering from it for more than 3 years. The method outlined in this book in the first chapter is extremely effective.

- Prime Publishing Co.

COPYRIGHT

Copyright © 2018-2026 and beyond by the Author

All rights reserved under International and Pan-American Copyright laws.
This book is revised and rewritten in 2026.

Book Title:	Reversing Insomnia
Sub-Title:	The Instant Guide to Sleeping Like A Baby Tonight
Author:	Rao Konduru, PhD (Also Called Dr. RK)
Publisher:	Prime Publishing Co.
Address:	720 – Sixth Street, Unit: 161
	New Westminster, BC, Canada, V3L-3C5
Website:	www.reversinginsomnia.com
ISBN #	ISBN 9780973112016

This book "Reversing Insomnia" has been properly registered under ISBN Number "ISBN 9780973112016" with the National Library of Canada Cataloguing in Publication, Ottawa, Ontario, Canada. The original manuscript has been submitted to the Legal Deposits, Library and Archives Canada, Ottawa, Ontario, Canada.

DISCLAIMER: The author of this book titled "Reversing Insomnia" assumes no liability or responsibility including, without limitation, incidental and consequential damages, personal injury or wrongful death resulting from the use of any treatment method presented in this book. Misusing the insomnia treatment procedure could lead to serious side effects. More specifically, overexposure to the bright Sun and/or to bright lights without appropriate caution and care could cause skin cancer, eyestrain or other health problems. All contents of this book are for educational purpose only and do not in any way represent the professional medical advice.

Dr. Rao Konduru's Publications	
1. Permanent Diabetes Control	www.mydiabetescontrol.com
2. The Secret to Controlling Type 2 Diabetes	www.mydiabetescontrol.com
3. Reversing Obesity	www.reversingsleepapnea.com/ebook2.html
4. Reversing Sleep Apnea	www.reversingsleepapnea.com
5. Reversing Insomnia	www.reversinginsomnia.com
6. Drinking Water Guide	www.drinkingwaterguide.com

The paperbacks (softcover books) and Kindle eBooks are available for purchase on Amazon.com for US residents, and on Amazon.ca for Canadian residents.

TABLE OF CONTENTS

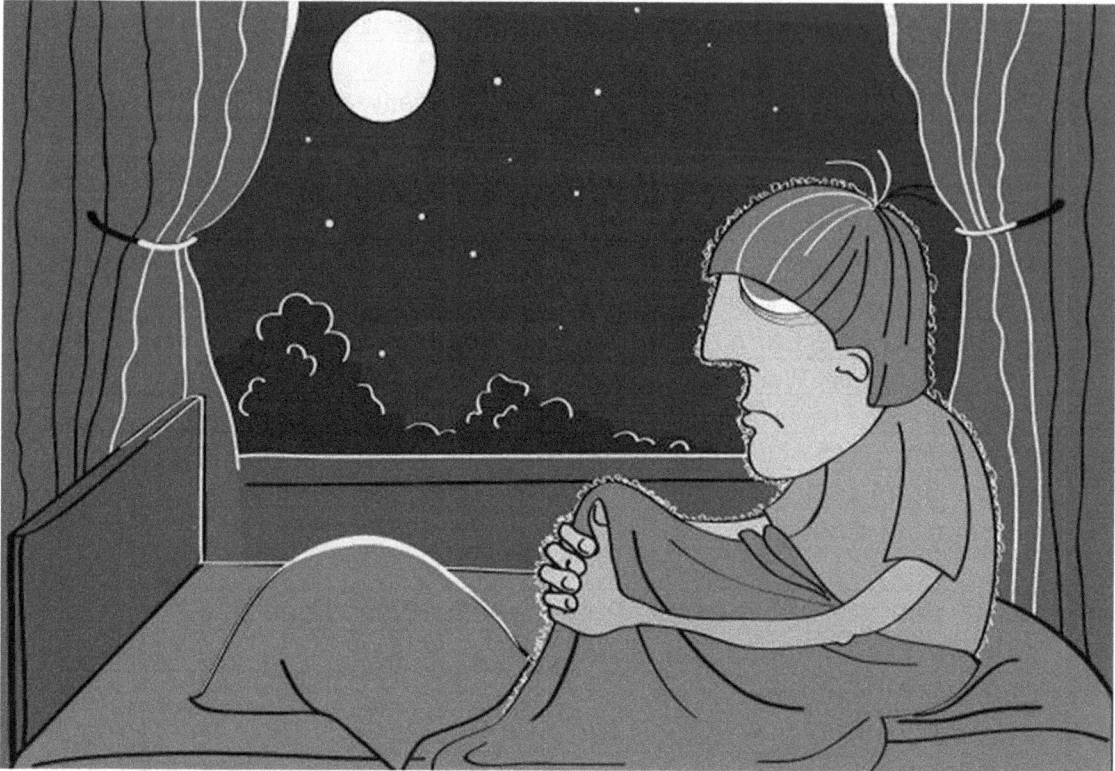

Figure 2 An insomniac is sitting on his bed awake in the middle-of-the-night.

Soon, you will be amazed to learn "how to sleep like a baby" by following the effortless and at the same time natural sleep method, self-discovered by Dr. RK who reversed his chronic insomnia in less than a week after suffering from it for more than 3 years!

IMPORTANT NOTE

CHRONIC INSOMNIA TREATMENT IS SUMMARIZED IN ONE PAGE, PLEASE REFER TO PAGE 10 IN THE PAPERBACK.

BY FOLLOWING THESE SIMPLE INSTRUCTIONS PROVIDED IN ONE PAGE ONLY (You don't have to read the whole book), YOU CAN EASILY REVERSE CHRONIC INSOMNIA IN 3 DAYS. IT IS ABSOLUTELY POSSIBLE!

However please read and understand the 24 detailed instructions of the full course.

CHAPTER 1: MAIN ARTICLE
INSOMNIA TREATMENT

INTRODUCTION

If you are suffering from chronic insomnia or sleeplessness, you most probably have developed the circadian rhythm disorder, which means your biological clock was disturbed and shifted from normal mode to the disturbed mode.

You have been staying up late in the night, watching too much TV, using desktop computers, laptops, tablets, iPads, iPhones, cell phones and/or other gadgets, spending a lot of time sitting under artificial bright light generated by fluorescent bulbs and LED lights, and reading on electronic screens exposing your eyes extensively to artificial blue light. This kind of activity tricks your body's biological clock into living a perpetual noon, mimicking the bright sunlight. Your body's natural rhythms would therefore be confused and your brain is unable to distinguish between daytime and nighttime. Therefore the pineal gland located in your brain fails to secrete natural melatonin that is needed to tell your body that it is time to sleep. As a result, you develop circadian rhythm disorder. This is the reason why some people fall asleep during the day and stay awake in the night, and feel the symptom of underlying sleep disorder called "insomnia."

If that happens, you need to reprogram your brain in order to reset the biological clock to its normal mode by making some simple lifestyle changes and maintaining the sleep hygiene outlined in this course. By taking appropriate action with willpower and self-discipline, it is possible and in fact very easy to reverse the circadian rhythm disorder in less than a week. Once your circadian rhythm disorder is reversed and your biological clock is adjusted and reset to normal mode, the hypothalamus in your brain signals your body to start producing melatonin, as is usual during the nighttime so that you would be able to sleep like a baby again.

In Order to Treat Your Circadian Rhythm Disorder, You Divide Your 24-Hour Biological Clock into Two Parts: "Daytime and Nighttime." And you should train your brain by informing it what exactly are the daytime hours, and what exactly are the nighttime hours. If you do so, your brain would understand your sleep-wake cycle, correct the circadian rhythm disorder, restore it from the confused state, and act accordingly to re-establish your sleep patterns through producing appropriate melatonin during the nighttime so you would sleep well.

DURING THE DAY	DURING THE NIGHT
◎ DURING THE DAY, YOU ESSENTIALLY LIVE UNDER THE SUNLIGHT WHENEVER YOU ARE OUTDOORS OR UNDER BRIGHT LIGHTS WHENEVER YOU ARE INDOORS.	◎ DURING THE NIGHT, YOU ESSENTIALLY LIVE IN THE DARK BY STAYING AT HOME. ALWAYS STAY INDOORS, AND DO NOT GO OUTSIDE. DO NOT EXPOSE YOURSELF TO BRIGHT LIGHTS.
◎ BY DOING SO, YOU WOULD LET YOUR BRAIN KNOW EXACTLY WHICH HOURS ARE THE DAY. For example 6 am to 6 pm, 7 am to 7 pm or 8 am to 8 pm. Each person is different so you choose your DAY hours.	◎ BY DOING SO, YOU WOULD LET YOUR BRAIN KNOW EXACTLY WHICH HOURS ARE THE NIGHT. For example 6 pm to 6 am , 7 pm to 7 am or 8 pm to 8 am. Each person is different so you choose your NIGHT hours.

If you live like that, within a few days, your master biological clock will be reset, and you will start sleeping like a baby thereafter. It works like a miracle!

CHRONIC INSOMNIA TREATMENT SUMMARIZED IN ONE PAGE
[By Following the Instructions Provided in This Page Alone, You Can Easily Reverse Insomnia]

You are suffering from chronic insomnia because your body's natural circadian rhythms and therefore your master biological clock disturbed, entered into a confused state, and unable to recognize and distinguish between daytime and nighttime. In that case, you need to reprogram your master biological clock. In other words, you need to train your brain and clearly inform your brain which hours are daytime and which hours are night time by doing the following exercise for a couple of days, or until you reverse your insomnia.

DURING THE DAY
a. During the day, equip your house or apartment with bright lights (no dim lights during the day howsoever), and live under bright lights. Go outside as frequently as possible, and walk on the street, and expose to the Sun while sitting in a beach or park. While walking on the street, look at the sky as frequently as possible desperately searching for the Sun. If the Sun is not visible, look at the sky and clouds. By doing so, you are letting your brain know that it is the daytime.

b. During the day, if it is cold outside, go to a shopping mall as frequently as possible, and walk in the mall. While walking in the mall, look at the ceiling lights as frequently as possible. By doing so, you are letting your brain know that it is the daytime.

DURING THE NIGHT
a. During the night, turn off all bright lights and live in the pitch-dark. Never go out and expose yourself to bright street lights after 7 pm. During the night, always stay home while practicing this Insomnia Treatment and until you reverse your insomnia. Finish your cooking and eating early by 7 pm or 8 pm, and turn off all lights, close all windows and curtains, and don't let the bright light from street lights enter into your house or apartment. By doing so you are letting your brain know that it is the night time.

b. **USE A BATTERY-POWERED LAMP DURING THE NIGHT AFTER 7 pm or 8 pm** while walking within your house or apartment, and turn it off while resting or sitting in the living room, kitchen or bathroom.
c. **You can watch TV by sitting in the dark**, but turn down the volume and turn down the brightness of your TV. By doing so you are letting your brain know that it is the night time.

d. After 9 pm or 10 pm, sleep alone in a pitch-black bedroom. Suppress all your thoughts, relax and sleep. Sleep on your side, not on your back (*Side-sleeping opens your airway, improves your breathing and stops snoring*). Let there be no noise howsoever, and sleep alone like a baby! **Please do not sleep during the day. If you are sleepy during the day, get out and walk (Go to a shopping mall and walk by looking at ceiling lights).**

BELIEVE ME IT WORKS LIKE A MIRACLE!
If you live like that, within a few days, your master biological clock will be reset, melatonin secretion will be restored, and you will start sleeping like a baby thereafter. You will start yawning excessively right from the first night. It works like a miracle, and you will sleep like a baby! Try it out!

This treatment plan is explained in detail in 24 steps in the following pages. Please read through all 24 steps, understand all concepts, and practice it. You will be successful!

INSOMNIA TREATMENT: PREPARATION
Please Follow These Instructions Strictly & Carefully:
1. LIVE ALONE AT LEAST FOR A WEEK TO TREAT YOUR INSOMNIA:
To try this insomnia treatment outlined below, you must live alone in a quiet place. You should not live with a group, too many family members, children and/or friends who make noise by talking loudly, or by eating and drinking, or by cooking meals and by partying under bright lights during the evenings and late nights.

2. LIVE IN A QUIET PLACE (NO NOISE) TO TREAT INSOMNIA:
You should find a quiet room, apartment or house, which is under your own control and where you could live alone without any disturbance caused by other people. There should not be too much noise. Your living place during the night should be extremely quiet and there should not be bright lights during the night. If there is noise coming from neighbors, you should fix that problem by talking to the landlord or you should move to a quieter place. You would essentially be living in an extremely quiet and dark place during the night.

3. YOU COULD LIVE WITH YOUR SPOUSE IF YOUR SPOUSE ALSO UNDERSTANDS AND FOLLOWS ALL INSTRUCTIONS:
You could live with your spouse only if the spouse would also follow all the instructions carefully, does not make any noise and would not live under bright lights during the night.

4. PURCHASE AND INSTALL HIGH-WATTAGE CEILING LIGHT BULBS:
Install high-wattage light bulbs (100 Watts) on the ceiling in all rooms (living room, bathroom, kitchen) except the bedroom in your apartment, condo or house wherever you live. These lights should dissipate light as bright as possible so that your eyes could stand and get accustomed to see the things around without any eyestrain. Usually 100 Watts light bulbs should do the job. These lights should have ON-OFF switches so that you could turn off all the lights after 6 pm/7 pm. By doing so you are training yourself to live under bright lights during the day.

5. PURCHASE A BATTERY-POWERED DIMMABLE TABLE LAMP TO BE USED IN THE NIGHT:
Purchase a few "Wireless, Battery-Powered, Dimmable & Portable Table Lamps with ON-OFF Switches," and place them one in the bedroom next to your bed, one in the living room, one in the kitchen and one in the bathroom. Many Dollar Stores sell these lamps. Most importantly when you get up and go to the bathroom to urinate during the night, carry the battery-powered lamp with you. Place the lamp away from you on the countertop and do not look at the lamp. Turn off the lamp as soon you get back to your bed or couch. By doing so you are training yourself to live in the dark during the night.

6. TURN DOWN THE BRIGHTNESS OF YOUR TV TO DIM LIGHT:
Using the TV Remote Control, Hit Menu button, scroll down to Brightness. Adjust the brightness by pressing the left arrow and/or right arrow buttons located at the center of the Remote Control. After you have adjusted your TV screen to the desired brightness (close to the lower end of the scale, that is DIM), hit the EXIT button.

7. TURN DOWN THE BRIGHTNESS OF YOUR COMPUTER MONITOR TO DIM LIGHT:
Press the BRIGHTNESS switch located at the bottom of your computer monitor or laptop. The BRIGHTNESS scale appears ranging 0 to 100%. Adjust the brightness to 30% using the up-down arrow buttons on your monitor. After a few seconds, the BRIGHTNESS scale would disappear, and your monitor would operate at DIM light.

8. INSTALL THE F.LUX SOFTWARE (FREE) ON YOUR COMPUTER:

Visit the following website, https://justgetflux.com/, download and install the software program called **f.lux** on your computer (**it is free**). F.lux makes the color of your computer's display adapt to the time of day, warm at night and like sunlight during the day. The program was designed to reduce the eyestrain during the nighttime and to reduce the disruption of sleep patterns.

9a. <u>Quit Alcohol Consumption:</u> If you are a frequent or daily alcohol drinker, you must quit before starting this Insomnia Treatment. Alcohol consumption mostly before bedtime causes insomnia at night and daytime drowsiness or sleepiness. So train yourself to quit alcohol consumption.

9b. <u>Take A Decision Whether To Drink Limited Coffee, Decaf, or Herbal Tea:</u>
Option-I: Consider Quitting Coffee, and Drink Herbal Tea Instead
♦ Overconsumption of coffee throughout the day disrupts your sleep and causes insomnia. For more information about how caffeine disrupts sleep and causes insomnia and chronic pain:
♦ If you believe that caffeine could be causing insomnia, and if you can withstand the coffee withdrawal symptoms, just go ahead and quit coffee. Consider switching to herbal tea. Organic Rooibas Red Tea has no caffeine, gives you energy and tastes good so you can easily adapt to it. Add some organic skim milk or 1% milk to it.

Option-II: Consider Replacing the Coffee with "Decaf Coffee"
♦ Please note that decaf is not 100% free of caffeine. The decaffeination process does not allow to remove more than 97% of the caffeine, meaning that 3% of caffeine is still present in decaf coffee.
♦ So "Decaf Coffee" presents an opportunity for you to consume a tiny or very limited amount of caffeine that could help keep you alert during the day.

Option-III: Consume Optimum Number of Cups of Coffee, Decaf Coffee or Both
♦ A person must research on his/her body and figure out by trial and error how much coffee is too much, and find out the optimum number of cups (1 cup, 2 cups or 3 cups) that could keep him/her alert during the day, and does not interfere with the sleep during the night.
♦ Under any circumstances, do not drink regular coffee or decaf coffee in the afternoon (be very strict). It is known to scientists that coffee could remain in your body up to 12 hours after consumption and could affect your sleep adversely, causing insomnia. So consume all the coffee you need (1 cup, 2 cups, or 3 cups) before noon. Do not consume coffee or any other drinks (Coke, Diet Coke, Pepsi, Diet Pepsi, or other soft drinks) during the afternoon or evening.
♦ During the afternoon, just drink purified water, ginger tea, or organic Rooibas Red Tea. Read CHAPTER 7 to find out the caffeine content of various foods and drinks.
♦ During this insomnia treatment as outlined in this course, even though you find yourself slept well all night long, you may experience afternoon sleepiness. In order to combat the afternoon sleepiness, and to remain alert throughout the afternoon, you should research on yourself and figure out, and consume the optimum amount of caffeine before noon.

♦ **FOR EXAMPLE:** The author of this book (Dr. RK) drinks 1 cup of organic coffee at 7 am when he wakes up in the morning, and then 1 to 2 cups of decaf before 11 am. That would keep him alert during the day, and doe
s not cause afternoon sleepiness or insomnia during the night.

FINAL NOTE OF PREPARATION: By following the aforementioned 9 instructions, you are preparing yourself to live under sunlight or bright lights during the day, and strictly live in the dark during the night. <u>Under any circumstances do not expose yourself to bright lights during the night</u>. This is the fundamental principle based on which the following natural method of "**reversing chronic insomnia**" has been derived.

INSOMNIA TREATMENT BEGINS HERE	
LEARN WHAT TO DO EXACTLY	
DURING THE DAY	**DURING THE NIGHT**
◉ As the Day Begins	◉ As the Night Begins
◉ As the Day Progresses	◉ As the Night Progresses
◉ As the Day Ends	◉ As the Night Ends

DURING THE DAY [7 am to 7 pm]
DURING THE DAY, YOU ESSENTIALLY LIVE UNDER SUNLIGHT WHENEVER YOU ARE OUTDOORS OR UNDER BRIGHT LIGHTS WHENEVER YOU ARE INDOORS.

As The Day Begins
10. Get up early in the morning at 7 am or 8 am whichever is convenient for you. Maintain the same schedule every day to get up in the morning and to go to the bed in the evening.
When You Get Up in the Morning:
a. Turn on all the ceiling lights (let all lights be as bright as possible for your eyes).
b. Turn on the TV (there should be some noise) and turn on your computer/laptop.
c. Walk to the window(s), open all the curtains, and look outside into the light.
d. Look for the rising sun and stare at the sun (if visible) for a few minutes.
e. If possible, get out of your home and look at the rising sun and sky for 5 minutes. If the rising sun is not visible, then look into the sky and clouds for a few minutes.
f. Walk to the kitchen, brew a cup of organic coffee or herbal tea (if you already quit coffee), and add a few tablespoons of 1% organic milk, and drink it.
g. While taking the coffee/herbal tea, walk to your desk, connect to the internet, listen to loud music on YouTube or listen to some music on the radio, check your emails and reply to emails, and turn on your cell phone, read and reply to all text messages, and phone all the important people and talk to them by making noise.
h. After taking the coffee/herbal tea, brush your teeth and take a bath, and wear office clothes and shoes (During the night, you are going to wear pajama and slippers only). If you continue living like that, your brain would recognize that it is daytime whenever you wear office clothes and shoes, and it is nighttime whenever you wear pajama and slippers.

By doing so, you are letting your brain know that the daytime has just started at around 7 am, and you want to remain fully alert and fully awake for the rest of the day till 7 pm.

As The Day Progresses
11. GO OUTSIDE AND EXPOSE YOURSELF TO THE SUN AND/OR BIGHT LIGHTS:
a. Every few hours (20 minutes each time), go out and expose yourself to the sunshine, which would boost your ability to sleep well during the night. Do not over-expose to the sun (that could cause skin cancer). If you do not see the sun, look at the sky and the clouds.
b. Go to a shopping mall, several times during the daytime, and walk there. While walking, look at the bright lights of the ceiling. By doing so you are letting your brain know it is daytime.
c. When you are at home, during the daytime, make sure all the bright lights of the ceiling are on in the living room, kitchen and bathroom. Try to look at the ceiling lights every now and then.
d. Never go into the bedroom, during the daytime, and never lie on the bed in the bedroom. Never take any naps by going into the bedroom or by lying in the bed. Bedroom is always a dark room that you would use only during the nighttime (between 7 pm and 7 am).
e. If you feel like napping or feel drowsy, quickly get out of your house or apartment and walk on the street. While walking on the street, look at the sun once every few minutes. If you do not see the sun, look at the sky and the clouds. By doing so you are letting your brain know that it is daytime, and you do not want to sleep.

EXPOSURE TO SUNLIGHT DURING THE DAY BOOSTS YOUR SLEEP AT NIGHT!

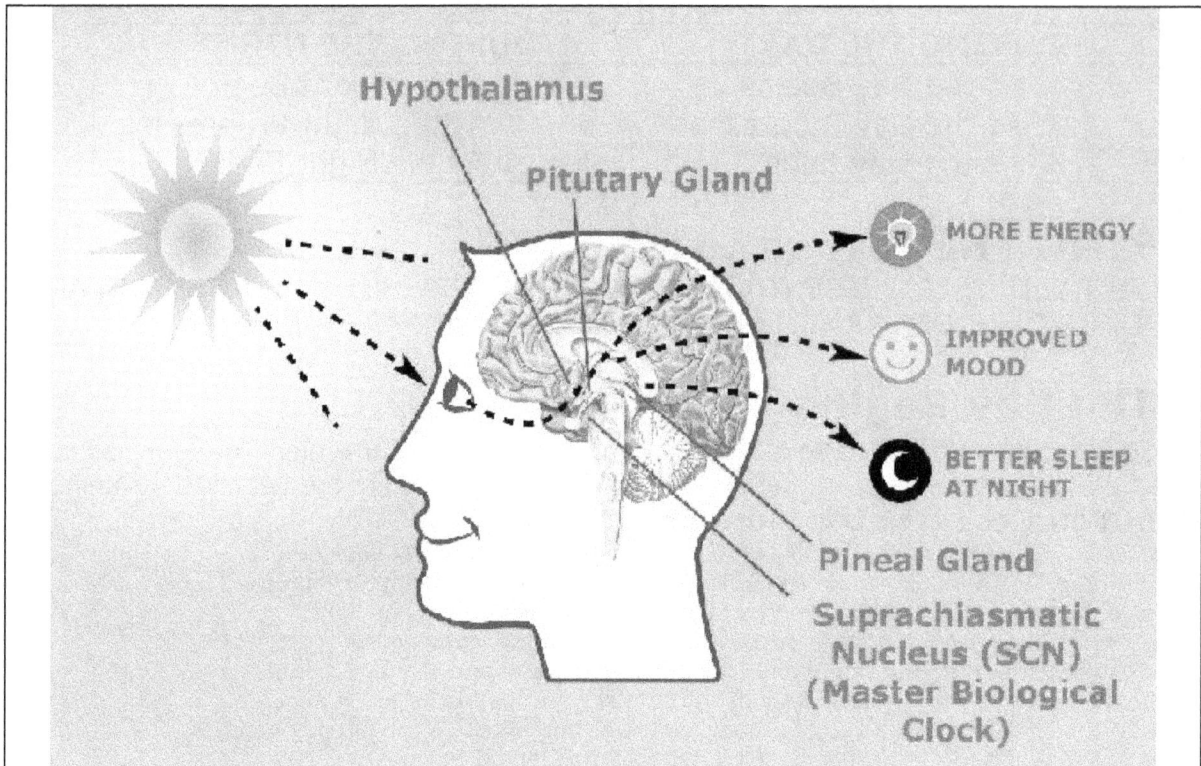

Figure 1.1 Exposure to Sunlight.

a. Sunlight or moonlight is sensed by the retinas of your eyes.

b. The pineal gland secretes melatonin at night upon the orders of the master biological clock, also called suprachiasmatic nucleus (SCN), located in your brain. The melatonin secretion is regulated by a rhythm-generating system located in the suprachiasmatic nucleus (SCN) of the hypothalamus, which in turn is regulated by sunlight or moonlight.

c. Exposure to the bright sunlight every day during the daytime regulates your circadian rhythm, provides you more energy, secretes melatonin appropriately, and boosts your sleep at night.

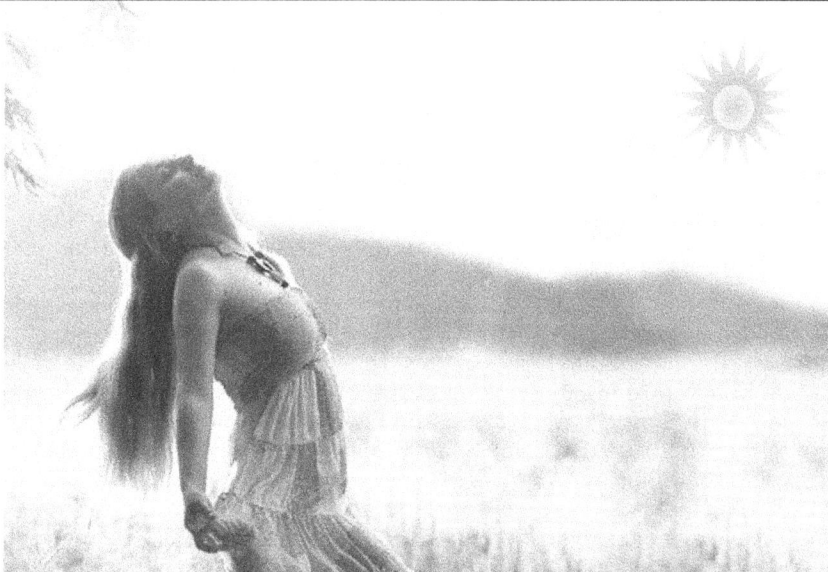

Figure 1.2 Exposure to the bright sunlight during the daytime boosts your sleep at night.

12. Exercise Every day

◆ Exercise improves muscle stimulation, reduces stress, and improves sleep at night.
◆ Exercise improves quality of sleep, gives freshness and improves self-image.
◆ Exercise in general makes you feel refreshed and helps you live with good mood.
◆ Exercise increases the efficiency of the heart and lungs, and keeps the body alert.
◆ Exercise on a regular basis also lowers total cholesterol & LDL cholesterol levels.
◆ Exercise helps you lose weight, keeps your body weight normal, and also improves your overall health.

You can exercise in the following three possible ways:

(i) You can go out and walk on the road (or street) for 1 hour, and expose to the Sun while sitting in a beach or park. While walking on the street, look at the sky as frequently as possible desperately searching for the Sun. If the Sun is not visible, look at the sky and clouds. By doing so, you are letting your brain know that it is the daytime.

(ii) You can go to a large shopping mall and walk there for 1 hour if the mall permits. While walking, look at the ceiling lights of the shopping mall as frequently as you can. By doing so, you are letting your brain know that it is the daytime.

(iii) You can go to a gym and exercise for 1 hour. You can run on a treadmill, ride a bike, do elliptical or other. After finishing your workout, go out and sit on a bench outside for some time and look at the Sun, sky and clouds. If the Sun is not visible, look at the blue sky and clouds. By doing so, you are letting your brain know that it is the daytime.

Burning calories can be accomplished through a variety of exercises such as walking and running, running on a treadmill, elliptical or biking in the gym, swimming, aerobics, bicycling, bowling, skiing, skating, stretching, playing tennis and other sports of your preference.

While any type of exercise would do the job, "walking, treadmill, swimming and biking" are most suitable and comfortable to most people.

13. Cook Your Own Meals at Home With Organic Whole Foods:

Do not consume processed foods and refined foods in restaurants on a regular basis.

14. Lose Weight if You are Overweight or Obese:

It is a proven fact that when your body resumes normal weight, your health disorders could disappear. If you are suffering from chronic insomnia, you most probably have gained weight. You must work hard to lose weight and make sure that your body weight is normal. You can find out your excess body weight and if you are overweight or obese by calculating the Body Mass Index (BMI) or by monitoring your body fat percentage. You should lose weight until your Body Mass Index or body fat percentage goes down to normal.

$$BMI = Weight (Kg) / Height (m)^2$$

For the complete weight-loss course, refer to another Book "REVERSING OBESITY (Self-Discovered Weight-Loss Method Illustrated)" by Dr. RK who not only reversed his insomnia in a week (in 3 days actually) but also reversed his obstructive sleep apnea by losing weight. Please visit www.reversingsleepapnea.com/ebook2.html for "Reversing Obesity," and www.reversingsleepapnea.com for "Reversing Sleep Apnea."

Given below are some weight-loss recommendations:

WEIGHT LOSS RECOMMENDATIONS (by Dr. RK)

Create a 2000-Calorie Diet (low fat, high protein) with organic whole foods only.

    a. Learn how to recognize whole foods, processed foods and refined foods.
       Eliminate processed foods & refined foods from your diet. Eat only whole foods.
       Stop eating out in restaurants. Start eating home-cooked meals made from whole foods.
    b. Learn how to count calories (if it is difficult for you, use measuring cups).
    c. Learn how to read labels when you shop for groceries. Eliminate foods with
       preservatives, artificial colors & flavors, saturated fat, trans fat, MSG, etc.
    d. Drink 8 to 16 cups of purified water every day.
       Do you know? Extreme weight loss contestants drink 16 cups of water per day.
    e. Take apple cider vinegar (2 to 3 tbsp) in a cup of water using a straw before meals.
       It acts as a hunger suppressant, improves digestion and promotes weight loss.
    f. Eat organic Kamut Puffs as a snack whenever you feel hungry in between means.
    g. Eat an omelet made with organic egg whites and veggies as a pre-workout meal.
    h. Exercise every day for an hour after eating the pre-workout meal.
    i. Minimize salt and oil consumption in all your meals.
    j. Sleep for at least 8 hours per night (If you have sleep apnea, sleep with the CPAP).
    k. Record your weight and waist size every day when you wake up in the morning.

Go on with the 2000-Calorie Diet along with daily exercise for 2 to 3 months.
If you do not lose significant amount of weight, then lower the daily calorie intake by 500 calories and continue for another 2 or 3 months.

  a. After 3 months, create a new diet by reducing 2000 calories to 1500 calories.
  b. After 3 more months, create a new diet by reducing 1500 calories to 1000 calories.
  c. After 3 more months, create a new diet by reducing 1000 calories to 500 calories.
    Do not try a diet below 500 calories.

For the complete weight-loss course, refer to another Book titled REVERSING OBESITY (Self-Discovered Weight-Loss Diet Illustrated) by Dr. RK who reversed his obstructive sleep apnea by losing weight. http://www.reversingsleepapnea.com/ebook2.html.

MY WEIGHT-LOSS JOURNAL: When I reduced my daily calorie intake from 2000 calories to 1000 calories, and stopped eating all junk foods (processed foods and refined foods), maintained high willpower and high self-discipline, my body fat (mostly belly fat) melted away. I lost 40 pounds and my body weight lowered to perfectly normal. When my body resumed normal weight, my obstructive sleep apnea automatically disappeared or reversed perfectly.

As The Day Ends

15. As the day ends by 7 pm or 8 pm, the night begins.
Read below the "Instruction # 16 & Instruction # 17 to understand
what to do as The Night Begins.

DURING THE NIGHT [7 pm to 7 am]

As The Night Begins
16. IT IS IMPORTANT THAT YOU SHOULD PURCHASE A BATTERY-POWERED LAMP. It is available in many dollar-stores for a few bucks.

Battery-Powered Table Lamp, Operates With 3AA Batteries

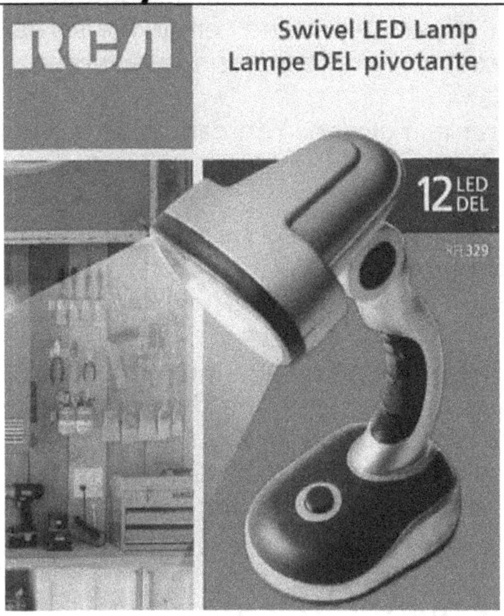

RCA Swivel LED Lamp
LED=Light-Emitting Diode
I purchased this battery-powered lamp at a Dollar Store for $5.99
when I treated my insomnia in less than a week.

SPECIFICATIONS
12 Super bright white LEDs.
Lifespan of LED bulbs: 100,000 hrs.
Swivel lamp head for directional light.
Operates with 3AA size batteries.
Can be used both indoors and outdoors.

It is capable to illuminate a small room with dim light. It has an ON-OFF button.

Figure 1-3 Battery-powered lamp.

17. DURING THE NIGHT, YOU ESSENTIALLY LIVE IN THE DARK BY STAYING AT HOME (STAY ALWAYS INDOORS) AND DO NOT GO OUT AND DO NOT EXPOSE YOURSELF TO BRIGHT STREET LIGHTS. YOU WOULD USE A BATTERY-POWERED LAMP JUST FOR WALKING FROM PLACE TO PLACE OR FOR DOING SOMETHING WITHIN YOUR HOUSE OR APARTMENT.

As The Night Begins (After The Day Ends), Do the Following:
a. FINISH COOKING & EATING: Finish all cooking and eating by 7 pm. Leave some cooked food in the fridge so that you could eat a little if you get really hungry in the middle of the night. No cooking and no eating dinner after 7 pm. You are essentially going to live in the dark.

b. WEAR PAJAMA AND SLIPPERS: Wear pajama and slippers as the night begins. Prepare to live under darkness after 7 pm as the night approaches. Whenever you wear pajama and slippers, your brain would recognize that it is nighttime, and prepare to produce melatonin from the pineal gland, later in the night. REMEMBER: You are going to wear office clothes and shoes during the daytime. If you develop this habit of wearing the appropriate clothes during the daytime and nighttime, your body and your brain would recognize and distinguish the daytime from nighttime, and will not shut down the melatonin production during the night. Melatonin secretion by pineal gland is the key to maintain sleep throughout the night.

c. TURN OFF ALL CEILING LIGHTS: By 7 pm, you should turn off all the ceiling lights in your house or apartment, and you should use a battery-powered lamp for walking and/or doing something for emergency purposes only. When you are sitting on the couch/sofa, and watching TV (dimmed at low volume), the battery-powered lamp should be turned off. From 7 pm to 7 am, all the lights should be turned off. Do not expose yourself to bright lights howsoever after 7 pm.

d. By 7 pm, turn off the computer, laptop and any other electronics.

e. By 7 pm, turn off your cell phone. Your cell phone should be turned off throughout the night. Do not answer the phone and do not read text messages on the cell phone screen during the nighttime until your chronic insomnia is treated completely and is reversed.

f. CLOSE THE WINDOWS: All the windows should remain closed. You can leave a window partly open for ventilation if you are accustomed to do so.

g. CLOSE THE CURTAINS: All the curtains should be closed making sure no light from outside enters your home. You should live in the **bitter darkness** at least for a few days, especially when you started this insomnia treatment.

h. DO NOT TAKE ANY KIND OF SLEEPING PILLS: Do not take any kind of sleeping pills as your doctor recommends during the night. They are unnecessary and they don't work exactly as they are supposed to. You brain is capable of producing enough melatonin if you let it know exactly when it is daytime and when it is nighttime. ALL YOU GOT TO DO IS: Reset your biological clock located in your brain by living in the dark during the night and by exposure to the sun and bright lights during the day.

i. DIM THE TV SCREEN AND LOWER THE VOLUME DURING THE NIGHT:
Dim the TV screen and lower the volume during the nighttime (7 pm to 7 am).
> You can dim your TV using your TV remote.
> Press menu button, press the brightness button.
> Adjust the brightness to minimum using the arrow buttons.
> Press exit key after you dim the TV.

You can watch TV during the night at low noise. You do the opposite during the daytime (from 7 am to 7 pm), brighten the TV and increase the volume. If you develop this habit, your brain would recognize which is the daytime and which is the nighttime, depending on the brightness of the TV screen and the volume, and produce serotonin and melatonin accordingly.

BY DOING SO, YOU WOULD LET YOUR BRAIN KNOW EXACTLY WHEN THE NIGHTTIME STARTED SO THAT YOUR SUPRACHIASMATIC NECLEUS (SCN) OR MASTER BIOLOGICAL CLOCK WOULD ORDER THE PINEAL GLAND TO PRODUCE APPROPRIATE AMOUNT OF MELATONIN ACCORDINGLY AS THE NIGHT PROGRESSES, AND MAKE YOU SLEEPY THROUGHOUT THE NIGHT.

As The Night Progresses
18. TAKE A HOT BATH BY SOAKING YOURSELF IN THE HOT TUB 90 MINUTES PRIOR TO BEDTIME:

It is the nighttime, and you are essentially living in the darkness in your apartment or house, and all the lights are turned off. You would be using a battery-powered lamp to walk within your living place from one room to the other. At around 8 pm or 9 pm according to your chosen schedule, one or one-and-half hours before going to bed, walk into your bathroom using the battery-powered lamp. Fill the hot tub with hot water, as hot as you could stand and get into your bathtub naked. Creating bubbles in the bathtub could keep the water temperature high for a longer time. You can enhance your hot-water bath efforts by using essential oils and/or the lavender, which acts as a sedative. Turn off the battery-powered lamp while you are soaking in the hot tub. Soak in your bathtub filled with hot water for at least 20 minutes by staying in the dark. The hot bath relaxes your muscles and releases any muscular tension that was built up during the daytime.

Your normal body temperature is 37 °C (98.6 °F). After you soak yourself in hot water for 20 minutes, your body temperature could rise to 39 °C (102 °F). When you finish the hot bath and get out of your bathtub, your body resumes the normal temperature 37 °C (98.6 °F). This sudden body temperature drop from 39 °C (102 °F) to 37 °C (98.6 °F) signals the brain to release melatonin, which tells your body that it is the time to sleep, but melatonin doesn't make you sleepy like a sleeping pill. It is your responsibility to put yourself into the deep sleep mode by relaxing and by living in the dark room. This technique works for some people and they become naturally sleepy after a hot bath.

After you have completed your hot bath, turn on your battery-powered lamp, empty the bathtub and walk out of your bathroom while carrying the lamp with you, and walk in to your living room and then to your bedroom. Then you would wear your nightdress or pajama. Then you should turn off the lamp, go to the bed quickly and try to sleep. If you are not sleepy yet, you can watch TV (dimmed at low volume) for some time, and whenever you start yawning or becomes sleepy, you can walk to the bed, close your eyes and sleep.

However you must always keep in mind that you are essentially living in the dark during the whole night. You would use the battery-powered lamp whenever you need to walk within your apartment/house, and turn off that lamp whenever you are not walking or not doing something.

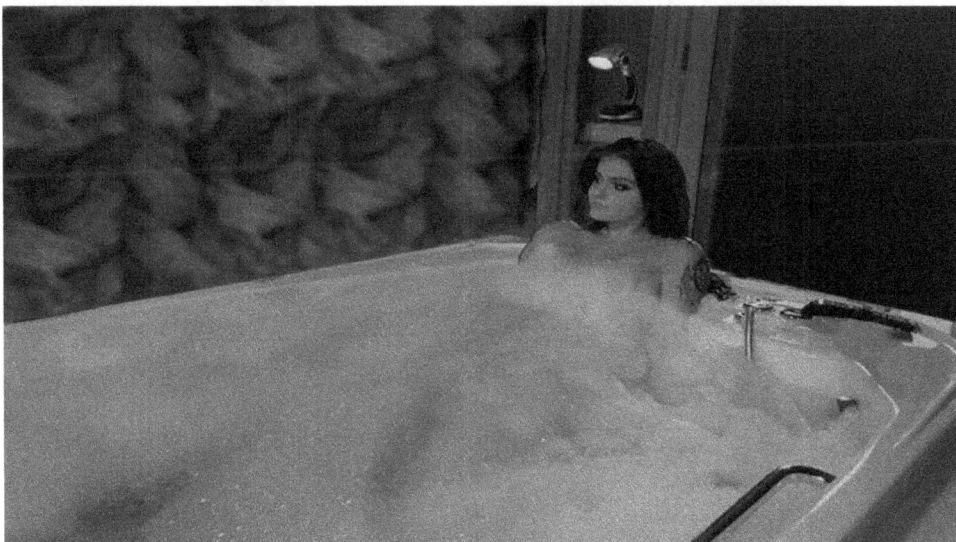

Figure 1-4 A lady submerged in hot tub (battery-powered lamp is behind her).

19. SLEEP IN A DARK ROOM (PITCH-BLACK ROOM) DURING THE NIGHT:

Sleep in an extremely quiet and dark room (pitch-black room), on a comfortable and cozy bed with nice pillows, throughout the night from 10 pm to 7 am. Wash the bed sheets and pillow-covers once every week or fortnight, and make sure your bedroom and bed are super clean all the time. No noise and no kind of light in the bedroom howsoever.

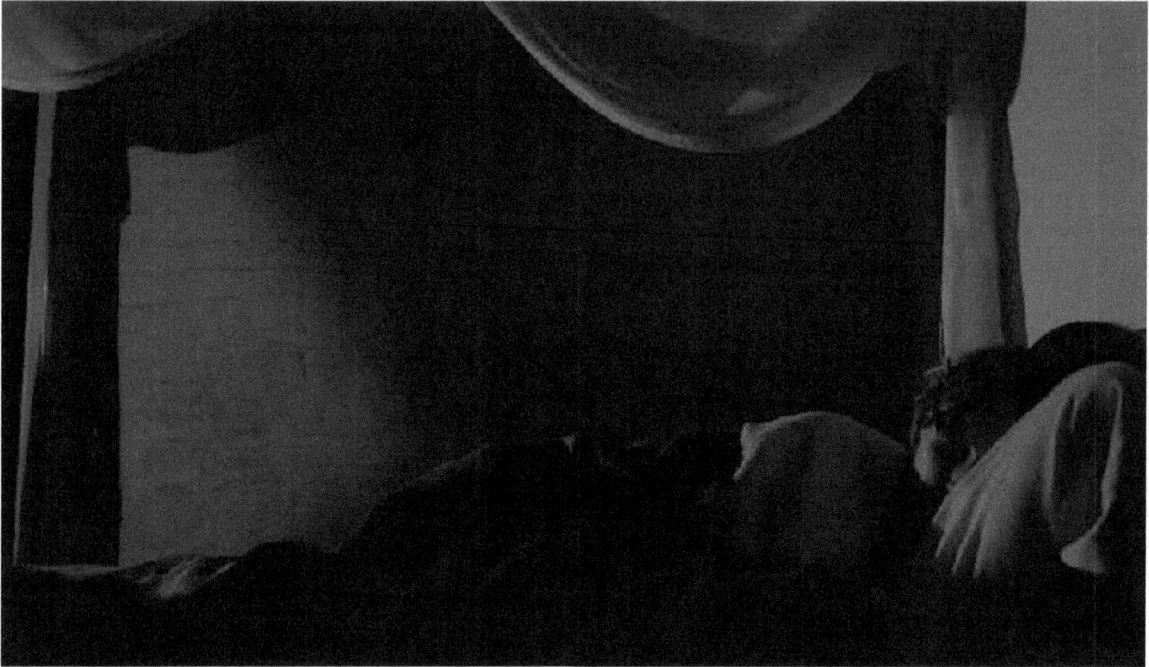

Figure 1-5 A person sleeping in a dark room at night (pitch-black room).

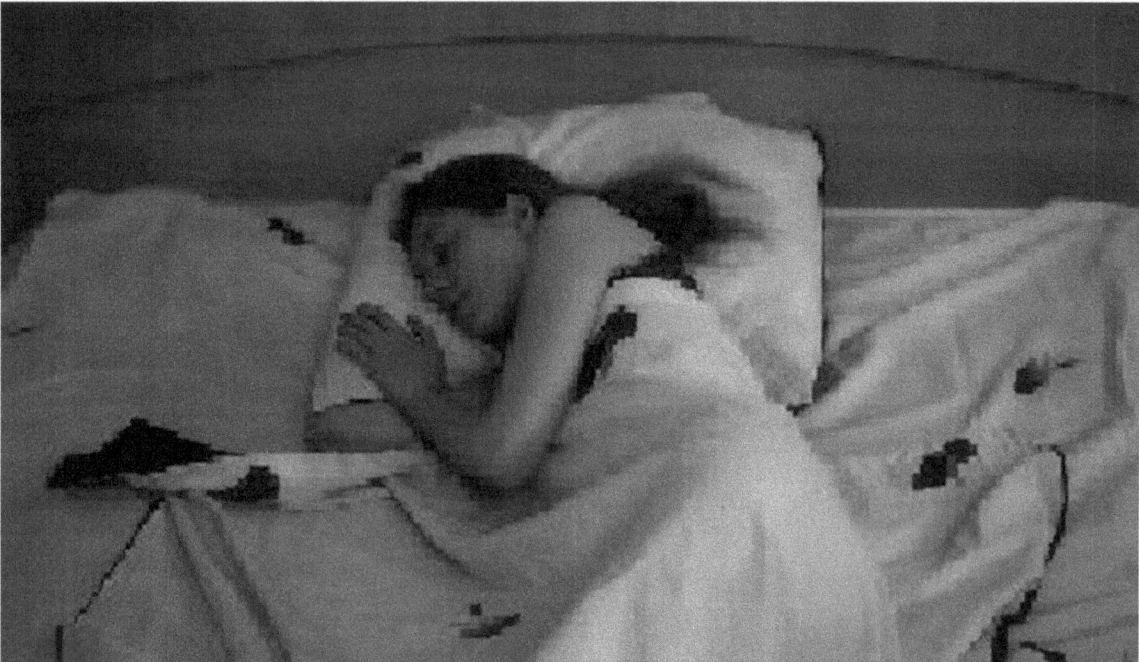

Figure 1-6 A person sleeping on the side in a dark room at night. Side-sleeping opens your airway, improves your breathing, stops snoring, and helps you sleep better.

20. TRAIN YOURSELF TO SLEEP ON THE SIDE (NOT ON YOUR BACK) [1]

When you sleep on your back, the soft tissue in your throat collapses and blocks the airway, and it is very likely that you could snore. Snoring could block the breathing, and the brain wakes you up frequently whenever your percentage saturation of blood oxygen (SpO2) levels fall more than 4% for more than 10 seconds. If the brain wakes you up too many times, that could become insomnia. You could minimize or completely stop snoring by sleeping on your side, instead of sleeping on your back. Side-sleeping keeps your airway open, stops snoring, and you can then breathe better and sleep better. So train yourself to sleep on your side throughout the night.

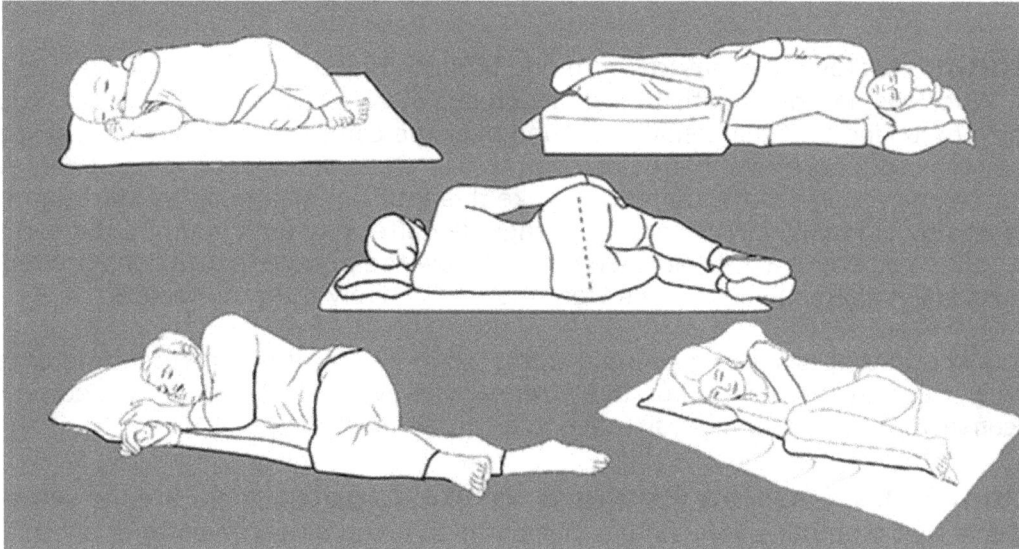

Figure 1-7 Side-sleeping opens your airway, improves your breathing, stops snoring, and helps you sleep better.

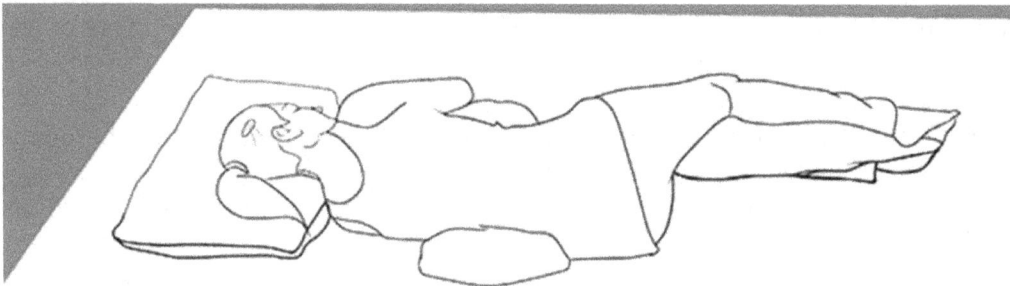

Figure 1-8 Side-sleeping opens your airway, improves your breathing, stops snoring, and helps you sleep better.

21. AVOID DRINKING WATER OR OTHER LIQUIDS AFTER 7 pm:

An adult is supposed to drink at least 8 cups of water per day. Drink all 8 cups during 7 am to 7 pm. After 7 pm, avoid drinking water or other liquids so that your bladder would not be filled with urine during the nighttime when sleeping. If you drink water or other liquids after 7 pm, you may have to wake up too many times for peeing and to empty the bladder, which could disrupt your sleep. However if you are accustomed to drink lots of water during the night, get up for urination, and get back to sleep without facing any insomnia, you can always drink plenty of purified water (RO water or distilled water).

22. SLEEP REMEDIES OR SLEEP AIDS

It is being recommended that you should try to reverse your chronic insomnia without taking any of the following sleep aids being sold in heath food stores, pharmacies OTC, or on the Internet without prescription.

These natural remedies are not guaranteed to work. They work for some people, and may not work for others. They may work for the first time, and don't work every time you use them. It is up to the individual to research on his/her body by trying them in all possible ways to find out if they are beneficial and if they induce sleep whenever needed.

a. Melatonin: Melatonin is a natural hormone produced by the pineal gland located in your brain. When the natural melatonin production depletes due to a sleep disorder, you can supplement it by taking artificial melatonin found over the counter without any prescription. Artificial melatonin is a hormone that helps control your sleep and wake cycles. It can help restore your sleep cycle at least temporarily. Take this artificial melatonin by starting from a low dosage and by gradually increasing the dosage day after day until you find the correct dosage that suits you and makes you sleepy. Also follow the dosage instructions printed on the label. Artificial melatonin liquid drops work more effectively than the tablets.

However it is known that artificial melatonin works when you try it for the first time or take it occasionally, but may not work if you use it repeatedly every day for an extended period of time because your body creates resistance to artificial melatonin.

b. Valarian, Hops, Passion Flower & White Zapote: These are the sedative herbal extracts that promote sleep. Take a dropperful in a cup of warm water or soothing organic herbal tea that is caffeine-free. [2]

c. Kava: Kava is a herb from the South Pacific known to help relax tense muscles. Kava was also found to be an excellent herb for relieving anxiety. Take a 200 mg dose of Kava extract standardized to 70 mg of Kava lactones. [2]

d. Calcium Citrate: Take a 600 mg of tablet or softgel about 45 minutes before going to bed. Calcium citrate is highly absorbable by the body. Calcium is primarily involved in slowing nerve transmission and in muscle relaxation. In other words, it has a sedative effect upon the nervous and muscular systems. [3]

e. Magnesium Citrate: Take a 300 mg of tablet or softgel about 45 minutes before going to bed. Magnesium citrate is highly absorbable by the body. Magnesium is an antidote to stress and a powerful relaxation mineral. Magnesium helps to relax muscles, relieves muscle aches and spasms, calms nerves, helps you fall asleep and treats insomnia. [4]

As The Night Ends

23. As the night ends by 6 am, 7 am or 8 am, the day begins.
Go to the "Instruction # 10 As the Day Begins," and read through to understand what to do as The Day Begins. As The Night Ends, The Day Begins.

24. HOW TO TREAT THE MIDDLE-OF-THE-NIGHT INSOMNIA

Please read through CHAPTER 4 for a detailed discussion on Middle-of-the-Night Insomnia.

Research proved that Middle-of-the-Night Insomnia is a very common and normal sleep pattern, and should not be considered a sleep disorder. So do not panic too much and deal with it by exercising calmness and patience. There is nothing to worry, our ancestors used to experience middle-of-the-night insomnia, and used to sleep in two phases every night. Sleep for 4 hours, remain awake for one to two hours in the middle of the night, and sleep again till the morning for another 4 hours. It is called segmented sleep, and is explained in detail in CHAPTER 4.

TIPS TO TREAT AND COMBAT MIDDLE-OF-THE-NIGHT INSOMNIA:

DO SOME OR ALL OF THE FOLLOWING TASKS WHENEVER YOU ARE ATTACKED BY MIDDLE-OF-THE-NIGHT INSOMNIA:

(i) MAINTAIN A REGULAR CONSISTENT SLEEP SCHEDULE AND MAKE SURE YOU ARE SLEEPING ON A COMFORTABLE BED AND PILLOWS: Go to bed at 9 pm or 10 pm and get up by 7 am or 8 am every day. Stick to this schedule and do not change it no matter what happens. Make sure your bedroom, bed and pillows are comfortable, clean and quiet. There should not be any noise howsoever during the nighttime. Invest some money in purchasing a nice bed and pillows. Always sleep on your side (not on the back), which would keep your airway open and minimize the snoring.

(ii) GET OUT OF YOUR BED AND DO SOMETHING IN THE DARK IF YOU ARE ATTACKED BY MIDDLE-OF-THE-NIGHT INSOMNIA: If you are wide awake and fully alert, tossing and turning, and unable to get back to sleep for more than 20 minutes, you should get out of the bed, and walk to the living room and sit on the couch/sofa for a while. It is important that you are sitting in the dark without any light.

IMPORTANT NOTE: Relax and do not panic, and focus on your breath. Do not let negative thoughts or past experiences come to your mind. Just think about the present moment. Breathe in, hold and breathe out. Focus on meditation so that all the thoughts are diminished. Or say some silent prayer, and repeat the same prayer over and over again, and focus on your prayer forgetting everything around you all the time until you become sleepy. Even if you are an atheist, you can meditate and say a prayer to nothingness or higher power. When you are really sleepy or find yourself yawning, go back to the bed and sleep. Or you can do all of the above while lying on the bed. When you are sleepy, you sleep on your side. Side-sleeping keeps your airway open and stops snoring so you can breathe better and sleep longer.

(iii) ALWAYS USE A BATTERY-POWERED LAMP FOR WALKING WITHIN THE HOUSE OR APARTMENT: Never turn on the ceiling lights during night from 7 pm to 7 am even if you are attacked by the middle-of-the-night insomnia. Stay in the dark throughout the night. Use the battery-powered lamp to walk to your living room, kitchen or bathroom. Do not leave the battery-powered lamp turned on for a long time. Use it only when you are walking from place to place and doing something in the kitchen or bathroom, and turn the lamp off when you get back to your bed or couch.

Leave the lamp on the countertop far away from you, and avoid looking at the lamp (You are using the lamp just for visibility). You can even watch TV (dimmed, at low volume) until you become really sleepy. When you become really sleepy or when you are yawning, go back to the bed and sleep.

(iv) PRACTICE RELAXATION MEDITATION: If you are attacked by Middle-of-the-Night Insomnia, get up and walk to the living room, sit with your computer desk, and practice relaxation meditation by sitting in the dark. Listen to binaural music for sleeping. There are many free videos on YouTube. Try the following video: https://www.youtube.com/watch?v=afEo2rxXAoM

When you have turned on the computer or laptop, and started the audio to listen to the binaural music (audio only), do not look at the monitor screen. Cover the monitor screen with a towel or cloth. When you are listening to the binaural music, focus on your breath. Breathe in, hold and breathe out. Focus on meditating so that all thoughts are diminished.

When you practice this kind of meditation, your beta state of mind would quickly switch to alpha state of mind, and your brainwave frequencies slow down. Meditation keeps your busy thoughts from intruding, and you become calm and drowsy. When you are really sleepy or find yourself yawning, turn off the binaural music, and go back to the bed and sleep.

(v) TAKE A HOT BATH BY SOAKING YOURSELF IN A HOT TUB 90 MINUTES BEFORE BEDTIME: If you are attacked by Middle-of-the-Night Insomnia, get up and walk to the bathroom, and take a hot bath in the dark bathroom (as explained above). Use the battery-powered lamp only to get into the bathroom and fill the bathtub with hot water, and turn off the lamp while you are soaking in the tub for 20 minutes. A sudden body temperature drop after the hot bath should put you in sleep mode. Your normal body temperature is 37 °C (98.6 °F). After you soak yourself in hot water for 20 minutes, your body temperature could rise to 39 °C (102 °F). When you finish the hot bath and get out of your bathtub, your body resumes the normal temperature 37 °C (98.6 °F). This sudden body temperature drop from 39 °C (102 °F) to 37 °C (98.6 °F) signals the brain to release melatonin, which tells your body that it is the time to sleep. When you are really sleepy or find yourself yawning, go back to the bed and sleep.

(vi) DRINK SOME WARM ORGANIC MILK WITH ORGANIC HONEY: If you are attacked by Middle-of-the-Night Insomnia, and if you are still not able to sleep, turn on your battery-powered lamp again, walk to the kitchen, drink a cup of warm organic skim milk or 1% milk with organic honey. Organic honey is soothing. Avoid honey if you are diabetic or inject the appropriate amount of insulin if you want honey. Milk contains L-tryptophan, an amino acid and precursor of both serotonin and melatonin, both of which promote sleep. Calcium present in the milk also helps you relax better. Get back to your couch/sofa, turn off the lamp, sit there and relax for some time. Focus on your breath. Breathe in, hold and breathe out. Let all thoughts be diminished. When you are really sleepy or find yourself yawning, go back to the bed and sleep.

(vii) EAT SOME LOW-CALORIE AND LOW-FAT SALAD WITH COTTAGE CHEESE AND DRINK A CUP OF ICE-COLD WATER: If you are attacked by Middle-of-the-Night Insomnia, and if you are still not able to sleep, turn on your battery-powered lamp again, walk to the kitchen, grab some low-calorie salads or fruits and cottage cheese (it is high in protein), drink a large cup of ice-cold water, and walk to your living room, turn off the battery-powered lamp, and spend some time on your couch/sofa by staying in the dark until you really feel like falling asleep. Be always in a relaxed mood, and don't think about your past experiences. All thoughts should be diminished. Breathe in, hold and breathe out. Just think about the present. When you are really sleepy or find yourself yawning, go back to bed and sleep.

(viii) READ A BOOK UNDER THE THE BATTERY-POWERED LAMP USING BLUE-LIGHT BLOCKING GLASSES: Blue light from the bright lights impedes your body's ability to fall asleep naturally because it interferes with the natural production of melatonin from your pineal gland located in your brain.

If you are still not sleepy after taking warm milk and after eating some low-calories food, and after meditating, read a health book or non-fiction book under the the battery-powered lamp by wearing **blue-light blocking glasses**. You can purchase blue-light blocking glasses on Amazon. When you are really sleepy or find yourself yawning, go back to the bed in the pitch-black dark room, just forget yourself, relax, and fall into sleep.

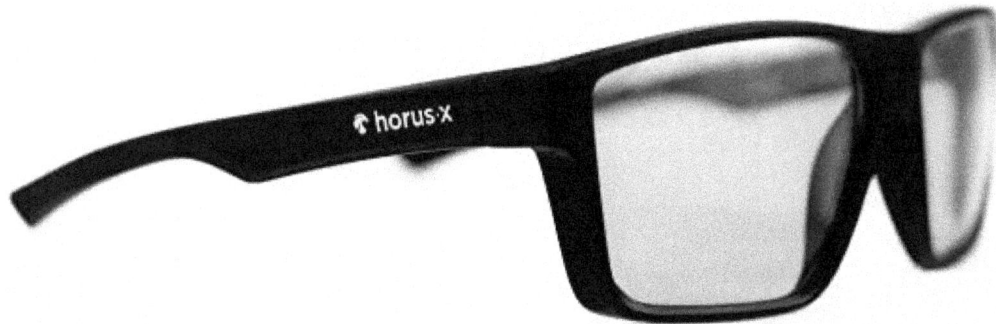

Figure 1.9 Blue-light blocking glasses (available on Amazon).

(ix) BONUS READING FROM CHAPTER 4
Middle-of-the-Night Insomnia Could Be A Normal Sleep Pattern

Don't panic if you can't sleep continuously for 8 hours (like you used to sleep when you were a child). You can divide the total length of your sleep into several segments, add those segments you have slept, and in average if you slept 7 to 8 hours a day, you should be happy.

SEGMENTED SLEEP: Segmented sleep, also known as divided sleep or interrupted sleep, is a sleep pattern where two or more periods of sleep are punctuated by a period of wakefulness. Along with a nap/siesta in the day, it has been argued that this in fact is the natural pattern of human sleep and helps to regulate stress.

During 1990s, an American psychiatrist Dr. Thomas Wehr conducted a study on photoperiodicity in humans to understand the sleep-wake cycle. He selected 8 healthy sleepers (8 healthy men) who were not troubled with insomnia at that time and who were accustomed to live in 16 to 17 hours of daytime and 8 or 7 hours of nighttime for sleep.

He placed them in a strictly organized quiet room. All 8 sleepers developed a sleep pattern characterized by two sleep sessions in two phases or two segments: All 8 subjects, when they were exposed to dark, tended to lie awake for 1 to 2 hours, and then fall quickly asleep. After about 4 hours of solid sleep, they would remain awake and spend 1 to 2 hours in a state of quiet wakefulness, experiencing some sort of INSOMNIA, and then they slept for another 4 hours. <u>Which means they slept in two segments: 4 hours in the first segment and another 4 hours in the second segment. Dr. Wehr also observed that there was a spike in their melatonin levels during the phase-II sleep or second segment.</u>

INSTRUCTION # 25
Light Therapy For Seasonal Affective Disorder (SAD) & Winter Blues

When you become unable to treat your insomnia by using the aforementioned 24 instructions, then you consider understanding and implementing Instruction # 25 as explained below.

Winter Blues
● In some regions around the globe, during the winter months, Sun disappears emitting no sunshine. Daytime could be shorter and night time could be longer. During this winter time, when sunshine is not available, the production of both serotonin and melatonin in your body is depleted, thereby developing either winter blues or seasonal affective disorder (SAD). Winter blues occurs in winter months causing sadness, mood change, lack of interest in performing daily activities, mild depression and also insomnia during the night. Winter blues can be treated with lifestyle changes with or without using any light therapy.

Seasonal Affective Disorder (SAD)
● Whereas Seasonal Affective Disorder (SAD) occurs in both winter and summer months causing depression, insomnia and even chronic insomnia.
● If you suffer from SAD, you may feel the symptoms such as sadness, grumpy, moody, or anxious. You may lose interest in your usual activities, and don't feel like working at all. You may gain weight as you don't sleep sufficient number of hours during the night. SAD can be treated with light therapy as explained below.

TREATMENT OF SAD USING LIGHT THERAPY
● LIGHT THERAPY needs a light therapy box or a lamp which can be easily plugged into the power outlet at your home, and can be turned on or off. The machine is built with either fluorescent lamps or LED lamps. LED lamps last forever and you don't need replacement bulbs. If the machine is built with fluorescent lamps, you will have to replace the lamps once every few years after they are burned out.
● Light therapy lamps are manufactured covering with a plastic screen to diffuse the light and to filter out harmful ultraviolet rays. So you don't have to worry about ultraviolet radiations that could damage your eyes.
● Light therapy lamps are manufactured to emit the light with a luminosity of 10,000 lux. You should sit close to your light box by maintaining 16 to 24 inches from your face for about 30 minutes every morning within one hour after you wake up. While sitting with the light box, do not look at the lamp directly but you should keep your eyes always open so that your retinas receive light with a luminosity of 10,000 lux, and signals your brain to produce serotonin.
● The light therapy machine is designed to emit a bright light that mimics and simulates outdoor sunshine, boosting serotonin, melatonin and vitamin D. Serotonin is produced in the skin, gut and brain and helps regulate the immune and vascular systems of the skin. The pineal gland of your brain makes melatonin during the night using some of the serotonin. If there is no serotonin available in your body, no melatonin is produced causing insomnia (no melatonin means no sleep).
● You should sit with the light box by maintaining the same schedule every morning. You can extend the timer longer than one hour, especially at night or on cloudy days. Please read and follow all instructions in the manual provided by the manufacturer.

CAREX Day Light Classic Plus Lamp to Treat SAD

The wider the screen of the lamp, the more light it emits to your face and body, and more effective the light therapy could be. Sit in front of the light box for 30 minutes every morning within one hour after you wake up. Remove your shirt and expose your entire upper body to the light therapy lamp. Do not look at the lamp but keep your eyes open. And maintain a distance of 16 to 24 inches from your face (follow the manufacturer's instructions).

Carex day light classic plus lamp is being recommended for best results. Please visit the following websites, do your own research, and purchase a lamp that suits your condition.

US Websites
https://carex.com/
https://www.day-lights.com/

Canadian Website (Resellers)
https://www.halohealthcare.com/
https://www.halohealthcare.com/carex-sunlite-therapy-light/

Sunlight & SAD Explained Here
https://carex.com/blogs/resources/light-deprivation-what-happens-if-you-don-t-get-enough-sunlight

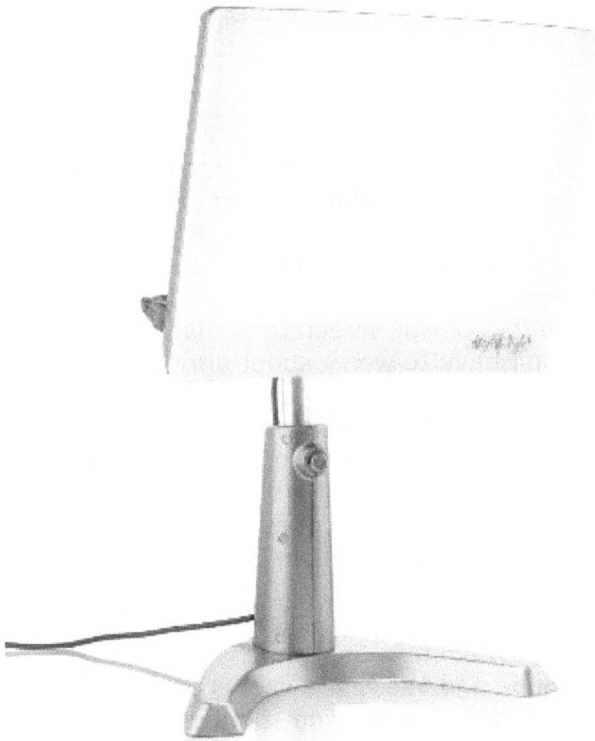

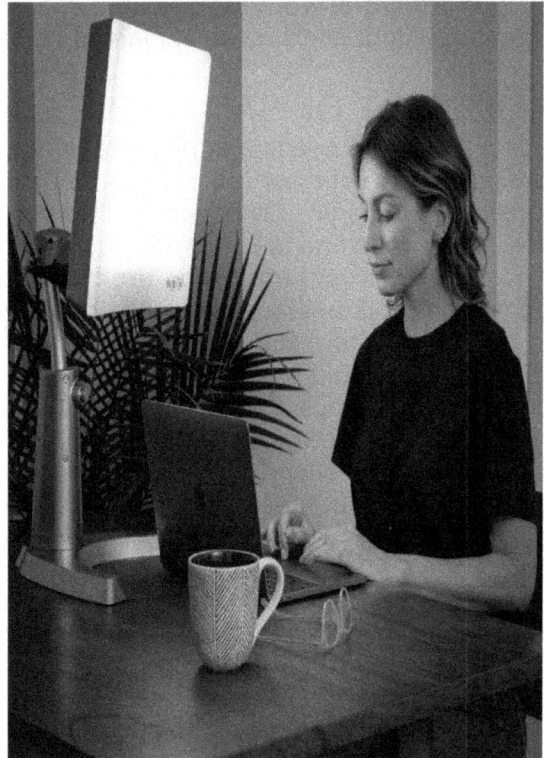

Figure 1.10 CAREX Day Light Classic Plus Lamp to Treat Seasonal Affective Disorder (SAD). Courtesy of Carex.

MEDICAL CONDITIONS THAT IMPEDE THE INSOMNIA TREATMENT

(i) CONTINUE TAKING ALL MEDICATIONS AND SUPPLEMENTS AS USUAL

Please do not discontinue your medications and supplements during this insomnia treatment. Continue taking all medications and supplements as usual.

(ii) VITAMIN-D DEFICIENCY IMPEDES INSOMNIA TREATMENT [5]

Research has showed that there is a link between poor sleep and Vitamin-D deficiency. Do a blood test and make certain that your Vitamin-D level is in the optimal range (over 100 nmol/L).
Blood Test to Be Performed: 25-HydroxiVitamin-D

RESULT		
	75 – 150 nmol/L	Normal Range
	< 25 nmol/L	Deficient
	25 - 74 nmol/L	Insufficient
	75-199 nmol/L	Sufficient
	> 200 nmol/L	Toxic

The exposure to the sunlight every day for 30 minutes to an hour would boost your Vitamin-D level naturally. If your Vitamin-D level is below 100, take some over the counter Vitamin-D softgels or liquid drops so that your Vitamin-D level is in the optimal range (over 100 nmol/L).

(iii) HYPOTHYROIDISM OR HYPERTHYROIDISM COULD ALSO IMPEDE YOUR ATTEMPTS TO REVERSE CHRONIC INSOMNIA [6, 7]

If your thyroid is not functioning properly, your body's chemistry would get out of balance, affecting circadian rhythm. Your master biological clock that is responsible for your sleep-wake cycle will eventually be disturbed, causing a sleep disorder called insomnia.

Two of the major thyroid dysfunctional problems are: (i) Hypothryroidism or underactive thyroid function and (ii) Hyperthyroidism or overactive thyroid dysfunction.

If you have hypothyroidism or underactive thyroid function, inadequate thyroid hormones are secreted by the thyroid gland, and as result some people may experience upper airway obstruction that leads to difficulties in breathing during sleep, developing both obstructive sleep apnea and insomnia. Hypothyroidism is usually treated with prescription medications such as Synthroid, Armour / Desiccated Thyroid / ERFA Thyroid Tabs, Cytomel or other.

On the other hand, if you have hyperthyroidism or overactive thyroid dysfunction, too much thyroid hormones are secreted by the thyroid gland, resulting in hyperfunctioning thyroid goiter, Graves' disease, or thyroiditis. This problem is usually treated with radioactive iodine. Several studies indicated that hyperthyroidism could also cause insomnia in some people.

If you are seriously suffering from chronic insomnia, you should also check your thyroid function by doing a blood test for TSH, Free T4 and Free T3 and should make sure that the test results are normal. If these test results are not normal, you should take the appropriate steps to fix your thyroid problem before trying to reverse chronic insomnia.

(iv) ELEVATED CORTISOL LEVELS COULD ALSO IMPEDE YOUR ATTEMPTS TO REVERSE CHRONIC INSOMNIA [8, 9]

A typical INSOMNIAC has elevated cortisol level, and cannot fall asleep or stay asleep and may stay in a state of arousal 24 hours a day. This can result in chronic insomnia. Even if an INSOMNIAC sleeps a few hours a day, that could be a very light sleep and is not at all refreshing. Some INSOMNIACS get used to segmented sleep. It may happen if you are living in a consistent state of stress, anxiety, and some health-related issues. Elevated cortisol levels impede your attempts to treat and reverse chronic insomnia.

Please do a blood test for AM Cortisol and PM cortisol, find out what was going on with your cortisol levels, and make sure that the results are normal.

The AM blood collection should be done between 7am and 9am.

The PM blood collection should be done between 3pm and 5pm.

You can take a natural supplement to treat your high cortisol levels. However you must fix your elevated cortisol level before trying to reverse your chronic insomnia.

(v) ATTENTION WOMEN! YOUR ABNORMAL ESTROGEN OR PROGESTERONE LEVEL COULD ALSO IMPEDES YOUR ATTEMPTS TO REVERSE CHRONIC INSOMNIA: [10]

When a woman reaches the menopause phase, the ovaries begin producing lesser amounts of key hormones such as estrogen and progesterone. As these hormone levels fall, symptoms of menopause show up, one of which is insomnia.

If you are being attacked by Middle-of-the-Night Insomnia frequently, it is likely that you are suffering from estrogen/progesterone imbalance. Do a blood test or saliva test or both for hormonal imbalance, and take appropriate steps to correct this imbalance so that you will be able to treat and reverse your chronic insomnia, and sleep well thereafter.

(vi) NUTRITIONAL DEFICIENCY AND MINERAL DEFICIENCY

Obviously any kind of nutritional or mineral deficiency could definitely impact your general health and sleep patterns, and may impede your attempts to treat or reverse your chronic insomnia. Please do a blood test to find out if you are deficient in certain essential and most common nutrients such as Iron (ferritin), Vitamin B12, Vitamin D, calcium, magnesium, potassium, phosphate and sodium. If any of these tests are not normal, you should treat and fix that deficiency by taking the appropriate high-quality supplement.

(vii) IF YOU ARE DIABETIC, CONTROL YOUR DIABETES PERMANENTLY [11]

If you are diabetic, you must make sure that your diabetes is perfectly controlled. Take the following blood tests once every 3 months, and make certain that all tests are normal. If any test is not normal, you should take the appropriate medications and/or supplements so that all tests would be within the normal range.

TESTS TO BE PERFORMED IF YOU ARE DIABETIC: Fasting Glucose, Hemoglobin A1c, Cholesterol Tests (total cholesterol, HDL and LDL), Triglycerides, Thyroid Test (TSH, Free T4 and Free T3), Prostate Test (PSA), Urine Test, Kidney Test, and Liver Test. If you are on cholesterol-lowering statin drug, you must take liver test once every 3 months.

If you are diabetic, please visit www.mydiabetescontrol.com, and learn how to control your diabetes in 90 days, and learn how to live like a normal person for the rest of your life.

(viii) CHECK IF YOU HAVE SLEEP APNEA [1]

Check yourself if you have sleep apnea by taking the "Overnight Pulse Oximetry Test." You can have a free test from any CPAP vendor in your area. If you have sleep apnea, you should sleep with a CPAP or mouthpiece or it could largely contribute to chronic insomnia. By losing weight, it is possible to reverse obstructive sleep apnea. So you should work hard to reverse insomnia. Or as long as you sleep with the CPAP machine, you should be able to live like a normal person, and sleep well. Please visit www.reversingsleepapnea.com, and learn how to reverse obstructive sleep apnea.

(ix) DO YOU HAVE CHRONIC PAIN, ARTHRITIS, FIBROMYALGIA OR MUSCLE TENSION?

If you have chronic pain developed due to arthritis, fibromyalgia or other muscle tension, it could also cause insomnia and impedes your attempts to reverse insomnia. So you should fix the chronic pain problem first in order to treat and reverse your chronic insomnia.

COFFEEINE CONSUMPTION GUIDELINES (by Dr. RK)
BONUS READING (Summary of Chapter 7)

● **Limited caffeine consumption has positive effects**. Each person is different! So each person must determine optimum number of cups of coffee (how many cups of coffee per day) by trial and error, and must drink all that coffee before noon.

● **Overconsumption of caffeine disrupts sleep, causes chronic insomnia, chronic pain, fatigue and other health issues**. Anxiety, insomnia, muscle aches, PMS (premenstrual syndrome), headaches, heartburn, and irritability are the other common symptoms.

● You should always keep an eye on every food item and drink you consume in restaurants and coffee-shops, as most drinks and some foods contain caffeine. For example, Coke, Diet Coke, Pepsi, Diet Pepsi and other soft drinks contain a lot of caffeine. Beware of the foods and drinks that contain elevated levels of caffeine, and keep them in your block list. Be cautious about caffeine content whenever you eat and drink out.

● Please do not take coffee or decaf in restaurants as the caffeine content there could be dangerously high. For example, Americano is loaded with too much caffeine. Do your own research and drink coffee or decaf at home.

● Research and find out exactly how much caffeine is present per cup of that selected volume of coffee you aimed to drink. Know exactly how much caffeine you consume per day by doing some reasonable calculations and by checking the labels of the coffee you purchased. If you do so, you can easily control the amount of caffeine being consumed per day, and can take action if you are affected by overconsumption.

● If you are too sensitive to caffeine, more particularly if you are over 55 years old with underlying health conditions, you better make your coffee at home from organic ground coffee powder. Stick to the same brand, stick to the same schedule and plan ahead by consuming optimal number of cups of coffee (1 cup, 2 cups or 3 cups per day to be determined by trial and error).

● Under critical circumstances, quitting coffee would be a great idea at least for some time. You can always get back to consuming limited coffee again. Withdrawal symptoms would last a few days, and it is not that difficult to quit coffee drinking. Try it out, you quit coffee for some time and you can re-start it anytime if needed. For example if you are too sleepy during the day, you need to re-introduce coffee or decaf again to keep you alert. Your own research would guide you and help you cure your insomnia and save your life.

● **Instead of quitting coffee, you can consume "Decaf Coffee" to avoid withdrawal symptoms**.
◆ Please note that decaf is not 100% free of caffeine. The decaffeination process does not allow to remove more than 97% of the caffeine, meaning that at least 3% of caffeine is still present in decaf coffee (in some brands, it could be a lot more than 3% of caffeine).

◆ So "Decaf Coffee" presents an opportunity for you to consume a tiny or very limited amount of caffeine that could help keep you alert during the day. However consume all that decaf your body needs before noon, and do not consume any coffee or decaf after noon.

CAFFEINE ALTERNATIVES

All kinds of coffee and any regular tea, including green tea, contain caffeine. However herbal tea does not contain caffeine. The following products are available in many heath food stores as alternatives to coffee. All these products, also called herbal coffees, contain chicory, which has some adverse side effects. They don't taste as good as some people say. It is up to the each individual to try and find out if any of these products can be used as an alternative to coffee drinking. You can purchase the following products in a local health food store. You can also try to find them on Amazon or by doing Google search.

1. Teeccino Caffe, Inc
   Santa Barbara, CA-93140
   Toll Free: 1-800-493-3434
   http://teeccino.com/

2. ALKAVA
   7298 Hume Avenue,
   Delta, BC, Canada, V4G 1C5
   Ph: 604-946-7277
   https://www.londondrugs.com/

3. Dandy Blend
   P.O.Box 446
   Valley City, Ohio 44280
   http://www.dandyblend.com/

4. Pero All Natural Beverage Coffee Substitute
   1455 Broad Street, 4th Floor
   Bloomfield, NJ 07003
   Phone: 973-338-1499
   https://worldfiner.com/

5. Organic Rooibas Red Tea (Herbal Tea, Containing No Caffeine), preferably taken with organic skim milk or 1% milk. It is being recommended as the best alternative to coffee drinking. It tastes good, gives energy, and you would be easily accustomed to it within a week after quitting coffee. Try It Out!

ENJOY ROOIBOS TEA.

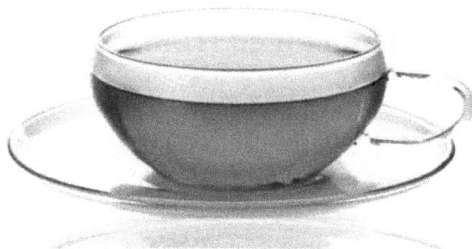

Figure 1.10 Rooibas red tea (100% certified organic herbal tea).

Rooibas Red Tea (100% Certified Organic Herbal Tea)
Best Caffeine Alternative (Milk Tea) Being Recommended!

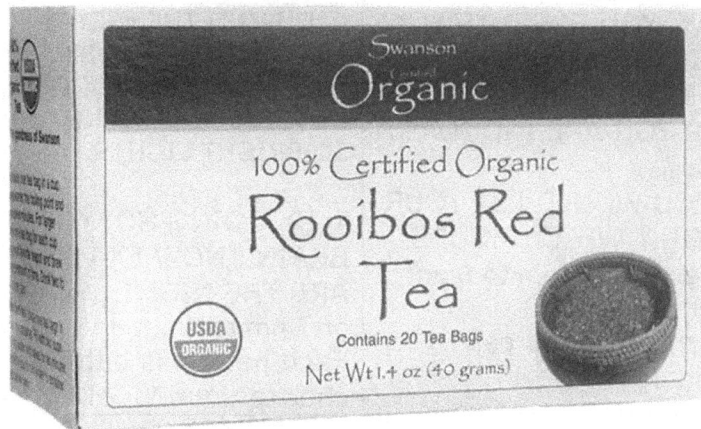

Courtesy of Swanson Vitamins
Rooibos Red Tea is available at www.swansonvitamins.com
Rooibos Red Tea (100% Certified Organic), Item # SWF082, 20 Bags, $3.99
https://www.swansonvitamins.com/swanson-organic-certified-organic-rooibos-red-tea-20-bags-s

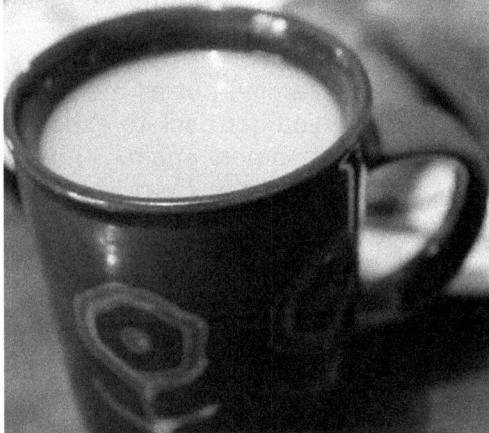

Rooibas Chai (Herbal Tea + Hot Water + Hot Milk + Cardamom)

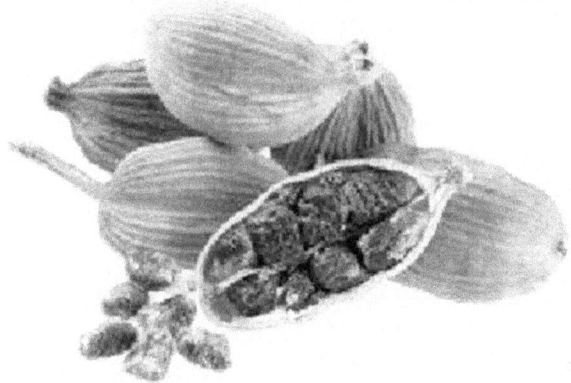

Cardamom Pods and Seeds

PREPARATION OF MILK HERBAL TEA/CHAI (Alternative to Coffee)
1. Boil purified water (do not drink tap water) using an electric kettle.
2. Add one-quarter cup of organic skim milk or 1% milk to a mug, and microwave it for 1 minute.
3. Place two or three bags of Organic Rooibas Red Tea/Ginger Tea/Other Organic Herbal Tea in the mug that contained one-quarter cup of hot organic skim milk or 1% milk.
4. Pour boiled water into the mug until it is full, and allow the tea from tea-bags to dissolve in the mug. You can press the tea bags to the wall of the mug by using a spoon. You will see the golden-brown color or chai color of herbal tea made from hot water and milk, as shown in the picture above.
5. Break cardamom pods with a knife and remove the seeds and add both skin and seeds to the hot tea in the mug, you will sense a delicious aroma and flavor while drinking the tea. Cardamom pods and seeds can be chewed as a breath freshener. Cardamom has many health benefits. Both the seeds and pod give a pleasant aroma and flavor. Enjoy the Chai!

Figure 1.11 Chai made from organic Rooibas red tea, hot water, hot milk & cardamom.

SUMMARY OF INSOMNIA TREATMENT

DURING THE DAY	DURING THE NIGHT
◐ DURING THE DAY, YOU ESSENTIALLY LIVE UNDER SUNLIGHT WHENEVER YOU ARE OUTDOORS OR UNDER BRIGHT LIGHTS WHENEVER YOU ARE INDOORS. ◐ BY DOING SO, YOU WOULD LET YOUR BRAIN KNOW EXACTLY WHICH HOURS ARE THE DAY (For example 6 am to 6 pm or 7 am to 7 pm or 8 am to 8 pm). Each person is different so you can choose your DAY hours.	◐ DURING THE NIGHT, YOU ESSENTIALLY LIVE IN THE DARK BY STAYING AT HOME (ALWAYS STAY INDOORS) AND DO NOT GO OUTSIDE AND DO NOT EXPOSE YOURSELF TO BRIGHT LIGHTS. ◐ BY DOING SO, YOU WOULD LET YOUR BRAIN KNOW EXACTLY WHICH HOURS ARE THE NIGHT (For example 6 pm to 6 am or 7 pm to 7 am or 8 pm to 8 am). Each person is different so you can choose your NIGHT hours.

IMPORTANT NOTES

● Be persistent, and do not give up after trying it out tentatively for a few days. Focus on the treatment, and try it out seriously, for at least a few weeks, by exposing yourself to the sun or bright lights during the day, and by living strictly in a dark place during the night after 7 pm. You will be successful in reversing your insomnia if you try it seriously!

● After reversing your chronic insomnia, you can live with your family, but all members should follow the rules for the rest of your life. BE CAREFUL! If you get back to exposing to bright lights during the nighttime, you may experience chronic insomnia again. So maintain strict rules during the nighttime, do not expose to the bright lights after 7 pm. If you live like that, you should be able sleep like a baby for the rest of your life.

SLEEP HYGIENE (General Guidelines)

Sleep hygiene is a variety of different practices and habits, a person implements by exercising high willpower and high self-discipline, that are necessary to have good night's sleep and full daytime alertness.

You Can Improve Your Sleep Hygiene and Can Reverse Insomnia:

● by exposing to the sun and/or by living under the bright lights during the daytime, and by living in the pitch-black darkness (always indoors) during the nighttime from 7 pm to 7 am. Watching TV (dimmed at low volume) is okay.
● by using a battery-powered lamp during night to walk within the house or apartment.
● by avoiding coffee, nicotine and alcohol consumption for life. Decaf or herbal tea is okay.
● by quitting all caffeine-containing foods and drinks.
● by taking organic herbal tea (which has no caffeine) with milk as a coffee substitute.
● by managing consistent and fixed schedule for going to bed and for waking up.
● by maintaining a quiet, clean and comfortable sleeping room (nice bed and nice pillows).
● by avoiding napping during the day (no naps between 7 am and 7 pm).
● by exercising every day and by avoiding the exercise within 4 hours of bedtime.
● by avoiding eating a heavy meal late at night (eating a light meal is okay).

INSOMNIA TREATMENT: How Long?

PLEASE REVIEW ALL 24 INSTRUCTIONS CAREFULLY!
AND GRASP ALL CONCEPTS OUTLINED IN THIS CHAPTER!

◉ If you read, understand and follow all the aforementioned 24 instructions carefully and responsibly, and if you exercise high willpower and high self-discipline without breaking the aforementioned rules, you should be able to reverse insomnia within a week. It is very possible to reverse insomnia in 3 days if you follow the instructions rigorously. Yes, Dr. RK reversed his chronic insomnia in 3 days after suffering from it for more than 3 years.

◉ Each person reacts differently to the aforementioned insomnia treatment. Living strictly in a pitch-black dark and quiet place during the nighttime is of extreme importance to treat chronic insomnia. Living alone during this treatment period could greatly enhance your ability to reverse chronic insomnia, as there would be nobody to disturb you. Do not expose to the bright lights under any circumstances during the night between 7 pm and 7 am. Use a battery-powered lamp only when walking within your house or apartment.

REFERENCES

1. Reversing Sleep Apnea: Proof that Sleep Apnea Can Be Reversed By Losing Weight!, Authored by Rao Konduru, PhD, April 19, 2018, www.ReversingSleepApnea.com

2. Caffeine Blues: Wake Up to the Hidden Dangers of America's #1 Drug by Stephen Cherniske, MS, ISBN # 0446673919, Book Published by Warner Books, New York, 1998, Pages 369-373.

3. Calcium by Dr. Dr. Lawrence Wilson.
http://drlwilson.com/Articles/calcium.htm

4. Should You Be Taking Magnesium Supplements? by Dr. Axe.
https://draxe.com/magnesium-supplements/

5. A vitamin D deficiency might affect your sleep. Here's what you need to know by Arielle Tschinkel, Insider.com, Posted on Feb 1, 2019.
https://www.insider.com/how-vitamin-d-affects-sleep-2019-2

6. Can Your Thyroid Gland and Thyroid Hormones Cause Sleep Disorders? by Brandon Peters, MD, Medically Reviewed by Elizabeth Molina Ortiz, MD, MPH, Verywell Health.com, Posted on March 03, 2020.
https://www.verywellhealth.com/thyroid-hormones-sleep-disorders-3014705

7. Thyroid Problems and Insomnia by Jon Cooper, Medically Reviewed by Michael W. Smith, MD, WebMD, Posted on July 15, 2021.
https://www.webmd.com/sleep-disorders/thyroid-and-insomnia

8. High Cortisol May be Causing Your Insomnia by Martin Reed, Patient Advocate, HealthCentra.com, Posted on April 22, 2015.
https://www.healthcentral.com/article/high-cortisol-may-be-causing-your-insomnia

9. Cortisol and its Effects on Your Sleep by Dr. Michael Breus, Posted on March 24, 2020.
https://thesleepdoctor.com/2020/03/24/cortisol-and-its-effects-on-your-sleep/

10. Can Menopause Cause Insomnia? by Kimberly Holland, Medically reviewed by Stacy A. Henigsman, DO, Posted and Updated on August 9, 2021.
https://www.healthline.com/health/menopause/menopause-and-insomnia#takeaway

11. Permanent Diabetes Control (book), Authored by Rao Konduru, MS, PhD, DSc, Reviewed and Endorsed by Dr. Marshall Dahl, MD, PhD, Faculty of Medicine, University of British Columbia, Canada, First Published in 2003, Revised and Rewritten in 2021, www.mydiabetescontrol.com

CHAPTER 2: INSOMNIA STATISTICS

TABLE OF CONTENTS

INTRODUCTION

Computers, laptops, iPads, iPhones, tablets, cell phones, many other gadgets, and bright light bulbs at home, work place, and outdoors, they all attack our eyes with "artificial bright light late at night," tricking our body's master biological clock into living a perpetual high noon, mimicking the sunlight. The master biological clock situated in the brain therefore enters into a state of confusion, and becomes unable to recognize that it is nighttime, and does not secrete the natural melatonin from the pineal gland, which is essential to fall asleep and maintain sleep at night, thereby developing insomnia.

I. 30-50% of The World Suffer from Insomnia: [1]

60 million Americans suffer from short term insomnia, and 30 million suffer from chronic insomnia. The numbers are gut-wrenching. Over 20% of Americans report that they have difficulty focusing on particular tasks, and nearly 20% claim to have mild memory problems, and over 10% report that they have difficulty in handling financial tasks. A recent survey found that nearly half of all Americans aged 65 and older reported to have unintentionally fallen asleep during the daytime in the past month. It could be due to chronic insomnia, obstructive sleep apnea or both. This problem is the highest among African Americans, who tipped the scales at over 52% having answered "yes" to having unintentionally fallen asleep in the past month.

II. American Adults (aged 18 and older) Spend 11 Hours A Day With Electronic Media (TV, Phone, Radio and Gaming): [2]

The average American adult spends nearly 11 hours a day with electronic media, according to a recent Nielsen report. A chart from the statistics site Statista breaks down our day based on data from the Nielsen Cross-Platform report (the chart can be seen in the reference number 2).

III. Info About Insomnia Statistics: [3]

◆ There are 40 million people with sleep disorder around the world.
◆ 95% go undiagnosed.
◆ 35 million people suffer from chronic insomnia.
◆ About 30 million have short-term insomnia.
◆ Only 5% will seek help.
◆ $100 million is spent in insomnia study.
◆ Around 1,500 car accident deaths occurred in 2008 around the world.
◆ 70% of insomniacs are depressed.
◆ 40% have anxiety issues.

IV. 95% of Americans Have Insomnia at Some Point During Their Lives: [4]

Insomnia is the most common sleep disorder in the United States. Chronic insomnia occurs in 25% of adult population. Chronic insomnia occurs in 50% of elderly population. A human being will actually die of sleep deprivation before starvation.

V. Sleep Disorder's Info: [5]

According to the National Institute of Neurological Disorders and Stroke, about 40 million people in the United States suffer from chronic long-term sleep disorders each year and an additional 20 million people suffer occasional sleep problems. In fact there are more than 70 different sleep disorders that are generally classified into one of three categories:
♦ Excessive sleep (e.g. narcolepsy)
♦ Disturbed sleep (e.g. obstructive sleep apnea)
♦ Lack of sleep (e.g. insomnia)

VI. Disorders of Sleep: [6]

According to the research, 40 million Americans were chronically ill with various sleep disorders, with an additional 20 to 30 million experiencing intermittent sleep-related problems.

VII. Sleep Study At Yale Medicine: [7]

More than 40 million people in the United States have a chronic sleep disorder, and many others struggle with sleep-related issues for which they haven't seen a doctor.

VIII. The Trivedi Effect: [8]

Over 40 million people in the United States suffer from chronic long term sleep disorders according to the National Institute of Neurological Disorders and Stroke.

What if there was a natural phenomenon that not only improved your sleep, but made your life more joyful and peaceful? There is such a thing and it is called The Trivedi Effect®! The Trivedi Effect® was founded by Mahendra Trivedi. He is able to change the very atom of living and nonliving materials with this energy. He connects people to the God of their understanding or the Divine Energies. People from all over the world and all walks of life have reported improvements in their sleep, greater abundance, clearer skin, greater intuition, better sex life, increased ability to focus, better relationships, increased self-confidence, more peace, more happiness, and so much more!

There are over 4,000 scientific studies that have been done on organic food, agriculture, genetics, cancer cells, viruses, bacteria, pharmaceuticals and nutraceuticals. These studies have been published in international peer-reviewed scientific journals. In one such study, Mr. Trivedi did a biofield treatment on brain cancer cells. After one treatment the cancer cells died while the healthy cells grew in size and number. The doctor performing the study noted that the Trivedi Effect® is the "holy grail" of cancer treatment due to its selective nature. Traditional treatment of cancer, chemotherapy, kills both good and bad cells, while the Trivedi Effect® only kills the cancer cells. These studies prove beyond a shadow of a doubt that the Trivedi Effect® changes everything at the cellular level! If it is able to change everything at the cellular level, imagine what it can do for you! The possibilities are limitless! To see more about many different scientific experiments visit Trivedi Science™.

IX. Insomnia Can Keep the People Underperform in Work, Costing the Employers Billions: [9]

Each night millions of people in the U.S. struggle to fall asleep or stay asleep. For some this is only a brief problem. But for others, insomnia can become a severe, ongoing struggle.
• 30 to 35% of population have brief symptoms of insomnia.
• 15 to 20% have a short-term insomnia disorder, which lasts less than three months.
• 10% have a chronic insomnia disorder, which occurs at least three times per week for at least three months.

Insomnia also can keep you from performing your best at school or work. One study estimated that an employee with insomnia loses about eight days of work performance each year. For the entire U.S. workforce, this adds up to an estimated $63 billion in lost work performance due to insomnia each year.

X. Insomnia Facts & Night Shift: [10]

Insomnia is not a sleep disorder in and of itself, but a related symptom of other problems, including an assortment of common physical and psychological disruptions in the sleep cycle. Statistics show that insomnia is a major problem among American adults. Approximately 60 million American adults report insomnia ranging from long-term or chronic to brief and temporary.

Symptoms related to insomnia are common among individuals that work night shifts or rotating shifts. Night shift work, while some people prefer it, is an unnatural human cycle. Studies have shown that this type of work over the long-term or in cycles can significantly disrupt your natural Circadian cycle. Interruptions in the Circadian cycle affects the physiological balance of your body and can vastly shift sleep patterns and inspire symptoms of insomnia and/or sleep deprivation.

XI. Statistics Posted by Sedca Ceutics LLC

In February 2013 a survey reported that 52% of Americans are losing sleep because they are stressed out. In 1997, a similar survey reported that 40% of all the adults said that they "lie awake at night because of stress." [11]

In August 2001, a scientist published a paper in the Journal of Clinical Endocrinology & Metabolism, reporting that the people with chronic insomnia had increased blood levels of stress hormones, and that that these individuals suffer from sustained, round-the-clock activation of the body's response to stress. [12]

XII. Statistics Posted by Dr. Paul Spector, M.D [13]

More than 30 percent of adult Americans, about 60 million people, complain of difficulty sleeping. For about a quarter of these individuals, treatment begins with medication (sleeping pills). This tells us two things: Sleep is a big problem and a big business.

XIII. Insomnia Statistics Posted by Better Sleep Better Life [14]
Insomnia Statistics Posted by Better Sleep Cottage [15]

Insomnia Statistics
- We now sleep 20% less than we did 100 years ago.
- About 40% to 60% of people over the age of 60 suffer from insomnia. Women are twice as likely to suffer from insomnia than men.
- Approximately 35% of insomniacs have a family history of insomnia.
- 90% of people who suffer from depression also experience insomnia.
- Approximately 10 million people in the U.S. use prescription pills or sleep aids.
- People who suffer from sleep deprivation become overweight or obese.
- A National Sleep Foundation Poll showed that 60% of people have driven drowsy. And 37% of them admit to having fallen asleep at the wheel.

Insomnia Costs Billions to Healthcare & Employers
- The Institute of Medicine estimates that hundreds of billions of dollars are spent annually on medical costs that are directly related to sleep disorders.
- The National Highway Traffic Safety Administration statistics showed that 100,000 vehicle accidents occur annually due to drowsy driving. An estimated 1,500 die each year in these collisions.
- Employers spend approximately $3,200 more on healthcare costs on employees with sleep problems than for those who sleep well.
- According to the US Surgeon General, insomnia costs the US Government more than $15 billion per year on healthcare costs.
- Statistics also show that the US industry loses about $150 billion each year because of sleep-deprived workers. This takes into account absenteeism and lost productivity.

These sobering statistics underscore the importance of enhancing sleep disorder awareness and why individuals need to seek immediate treatment for the health and well-being of others.

XIV. Insomnia Statistics Posted by Sleep and Sleep Disorder Statistics, American Sleep Association [16]

- 50-70 Million US adults have some kind of sleep disorder and 48% snore.
- 37.9% reported unintentionally falling asleep during the day.
- 4.7% reported nodding off or falling asleep while driving.
- Drowsy driving is the reason for 1,550 fatalities and 40,000 non-fatal injuries annually in the United States alone.
- 100,000 deaths occur each year in US hospitals due to medical errors and sleep deprivation has been shown to make a significant contribution.
- Insomnia is the most common sleep disorder, with short-term issues reported by about 30% of adults and chronic insomnia by 10%.
- 3–5% of the obese adults could be attributable to short sleep.
- 37% of 20-39 year-olds report short sleep duration.
- 40% of 40-59 year-olds report short sleep duration.
- 35.3% adults report < 7 hours of sleep during a typical 24-hour period.

How Many Hours of Sleep Do People Need? [16]
[American Sleep Association]

Infants 4 -12 months:	12 – 16 hours (including naps)
Children (Ages 1 – 2 years)	11 – 14 hours (including naps)
Children (Ages 3 – 5 years)	10 – 13 hours (including naps)
Children (Ages 6 – 12 years)	9 - 12 hours
Teenagers	8 – 10 hours
Adults	7 – 9 hours

XV. Insomnia Statistics Posted by Brain Research Institute [17]

- 40 Million people in the U.S. have a chronic sleep disorder.
- Estimated cost to U.S. employers in lost productivity = $18 Billion.
- 62% of American adults experience a sleep problem a few nights per week.
- 30% of all adults have insomnia in the course of any year.
- 31% of high school students reported getting an average of at least 8 hours.

How Many Hours of Sleep Do People Need? [17]
[Brain Research Institute]

Children (Ages 5 – 10)	11 hours
Teenagers (Ages 10 – 17)	9 hours
Adults	8 hours

XVI. Insomnia Statistics Posted by Warwick University [18]

♦ Global 'Sleeplessness Epidemic' Affects an estimated 150 million sufferers in the developing world. The survey undertook in eight locations of rural populations in Ghana, Tanzania, South Africa, India, Bangladesh, Vietnam and Indonesia, and an urban area in Kenya.

♦ Bangladesh had the highest prevalence of sleep problems among the countries analyzed – with a 43.9% rate for women – more than twice the rate of developed countries and far higher than the 23.6% seen in men. Bangladesh also saw very high patterns of anxiety and depression.

♦ Vietnam too had very high rates of sleep problems 37.6% for women and 28.5% for men.

♦ Meanwhile in African countries, Tanzania, Kenya and Ghana, the rates are between 8.3% and 12.7%.

♦ However South Africa had double the rate of the other African countries – 31.3% for women and 27.2% for men.

♦ India and Indonesia both had very low prevalence of sleep issues – 6.5% for Indian women and 4.3% for Indian men. Indonesian men reported rates of sleep problems of 3.9$ and women had rates of 4.6%.

XVII. INSOMNIA STATISTICS Posted by Statistics Canada [19, 20]

♦ In 2002 an estimated 3.3 million Canadians aged 15 or older had insomnia. Canadian Community Health Survey (CCHS) found that 18% of these people sleep less than five hours a night.

♦ The study found that stress and chronic conditions such as arthritis that involves pain causes insomnia.

♦ The study showed that middle-aged people (ages 45 to 64) had high odds of suffering from insomnia, as did people who were widowed and people with low education.

♦ Weight gain is a contributing factor in causing insomnia. High proportions of people who were obese suffered from insomnia. The heavier they were, the more likely they were to have trouble sleeping. The study also found that heavy weekly drinking was linked to insomnia, as was frequent use of cannabis (a street drug).

♦ People aged 45 to 64 had significantly higher odds of reporting insomnia compared with those aged 15 to 24.

XVIII. INSOMNIA STATISTICS Posted by CBC News Health [21]

♦ Recent research indicates 35 per cent of Canadian youth aged 12 to 17 and 61 per cent of adults get fewer than eight hours of sleep a night.

♦ Too often, not getting enough sleep is seen as badge of honor in our society, Dr. Charles Samuels of the Canadian Sleep Society said.

♦ Recent research indicates 35% of Canadian youth aged 12 to 17, and 61% of adults get fewer than eight hours of sleep a night.

♦ Insomnia, obstructive sleep apnea, restless legs syndrome and sleep deprivation in general affect up to 45% of the world's population, the World Association of Sleep Medicine said in a report released to mark the organization's 2011 World Sleep Day.

♦ Women have a higher rate of trouble falling asleep and staying asleep — 35% compared with 25% for men.

♦ A person who has not slept for 20 hours has a level of impairment equivalent to someone with a blood alcohol concentration of 0.08%, over the limit of 0.05%, at which a driver is considered legally impaired in Ontario.

♦ A non-typical sleep schedule from shift work disturbs the body's natural pattern of rest and rejuvenation, which can lead to physical and mental problems, including cardiovascular disease, hypertension, asthma, diabetes and depression.

♦Chronic sleep deprivation can contribute to obesity, diabetes, high blood pressure, heart attack, stroke and other medical conditions. The amount of sleep and the quality of sleep have been shown to affect appetite, weight control and the effectiveness of diets for weight loss.

♦ An extra hour of sleep at night appears to decrease the risk of coronary heart calcification, or hardening of the arteries, an early indicator of cardiovascular disease.

♦ Poor sleep affects about 25% of the world's children, according to the sleep medicine group.

♦ As many as 40% of [Canadian] children aren't getting enough sleep, which is not only impairing their ability to function properly, it is hurting their ability to learn.

♦ Doctors suggest teenagers need about 9 hours of sleep a night. Children in elementary school should be getting 10 to 12 hours.

XIX. INSOMNIA & INSOMNIA STATISTICS
Posted by Lundbeck (Beijing) Pharmaceutical Consulting Co, Ltd. [22]

♦ Insomnia is the most common sleep disorder, chronically affecting approximately 10–15% of the population. The risk of insomnia increases with age;
A US study revealed that 29% of adults aged over 65 years have insomnia.

The prevalence of sleeping problems varies with geographic location:
56% of people in the US,
31% in Western Europe, and
23% in Japan have reported difficulty in sleeping

♦ A Canadian study estimated that insomnia costs approximately $5,000 per person every year. Most of this cost was due to reduced productivity at work (76%) and absenteeism (15%).

♦ Very few people suffering from insomnia go to see a doctor, making it an under-diagnosed and under-treated disorder. In a European survey, it was found that 37% of people with insomnia took no action to resolve it at all, 10% used over-the-counter remedies and 13% adopted non-pharmacological measures.

♦Insomnia can be treated with a combination of sleep hygiene, cognitive behavioral therapy and medication. Sleep hygiene covers topics such as establishing a sleep routine, exercising frequently and avoiding lying awake in bed. Various behavioral therapies can also be used, such as relaxation, postponing bedtime and sleep restriction.

XX. INSOMNIA STATISTICS:
A List of 16 Eye-Opening Stats/Facts
by Candace Osmond at Sleep Judge [23]

#1. Women Suffer from Insomnia Worse Than Men.
#2. More Than Half of all Americans are Regularly Losing Sleep Because They Are Worrying.
#3. Insomnia is More Common Than You Think.
#4. If You Suffer from Depression, You Are Also Likely to Find It Difficult to Sleep.
#5. Alternative Treatments Can Help Alleviate Insomnia.
#6. Napping Can Cause Insomnia.
#7. There is a Link Between Insomnia and Weight Gain.
#8. More Than 10 Million People Are Regularly Taking Sleeping Pills.
#9. Staying Up Late Can Trigger Insomnia.
#10. Alcohol Can Disrupt Your Sleep Pattern.
#11. There Are Three Types of Insomnia.
#12. Thousands of People Are Driving While Sleepy.
#13. Lack of Sleep Can Have a Serious Impact on Your Relationships.
#14. People Sleep Less Now Than a Century Ago.
#15. Caffeine is Not Your Friend.
#16. Insomnia Has a Financial Impact on Healthcare & Employers.

XXI. 7 Strange Facts About Insomnia [24]

#1. Insomnia can be hereditary.
#2. Pets and bugs can also suffer from insomnia.
#3. Social jet lag can be a drag.
#4. Sleeping pills are still popular, despite their failure to cure insomnia.
#5. Women's hormones may play a role in insomnia.
#6. In rare cases, people can die from insomnia.
#7. Chronic insomnia, if left untreated, increases the risk of alcohol abuse.

XXII. INSOMNIA STATISTICS BY COUNTRY,
Posted by RightDiagnosis.com, 2004 [25]

RightDiagnosis.com is one of the world's leading providers of online medical health information. The site is an independent, objective source for factual, mainstream health information for both consumers and health professionals.

The following table attempts to extrapolate the above prevalence rate for Insomnia to the populations of various countries and regions. These prevalence extrapolations for Insomnia are only estimates, based on applying the prevalence rates from the US (or a similar country) to the population of other countries, and therefore may have very limited relevance to the actual prevalence of Insomnia in any region.

The following country-wise insomnia statistics show the name of the country, population in 2004, and the number of insomnia sufferers in each country in 2004:

Table 2.1 Insomnia statistics by country.

Country	Population	Insomnia Sufferers
USA	293,655,405	34,547,694
Canada	32,507,874	3,824,455
Mexico	104,959,594	12,348,187
Brazil	184,101,109	21,658,953
UK	60,270,708	7,090,671
France	60,424,213	7,108,730
India	1,065,070,607	125,302,421
China	1,298,847,624	152,805,599
Japan	127,333,002	14,980,352

For the insomnia statistics of other countries, visit the website:
http://www.rightdiagnosis.com/i/insomnia/stats-country.htm

XXIII. THE PREVALENCE OF INSOMNIA EXPLAINED IN JOURNAL PUBLICATIONS [26, 27, 28, 29]

The following journal publications discuss in detail about the country-wise prevalence of insomnia and about the insomnia statistics (see references):
a. Epidemiology of insomnia: A review of the Global and Indian scenario
b. Prevalence of insomnia among Chinese adults in Hong Kong: a population-based study
c. Epidemiology of Insomnia, Prevalence and Risk Factors
d. Prevalence of Insomnia in Europe: A Comparison of 6 Countries

REFERENCES

1. Living with Chronic Insomnia: A Living Hell by Admin, The Original Miracle Wedge.
http://www.miraclewedgepillow.com/sleep-apnea/chronic-insomnia-a-living-hell/

2. American Adults (18+) Spend 11 Hours A Day With Electronic Media (TV, Phone, Radio and Gaming).
http://time.com/16458/nielsen-electronic-media-study-11-hours-a-day/

3. Info About Insomnia (Slide 19), Slide Show by Melvin Hernandez.
https://www.slideshare.net/melvinhernandez/insomnia-2615230

4. Insomnia is the Most Common Sleep Disorder in US, Daniel Lyons @NutraRelief.
https://twitter.com/nutrarelief

5. Sleep Disorder's Info.
http://www.ussleeplab.com/sleep-disorders-info/

6. Disorders of Sleep: An overview, Leon Ting, MD and Atul Malhotra, MD.
https://www.ncbi.nlm.nih.gov/pmc/articles/PMC4368182/

7. Sleep Study: Yale Medicine.
https://www.yalemedicine.org/conditions/sleep-study/

8. Got Sleep?
https://www.trivedieffect.com/inspiration-blog/got-sleep/

9. Insomnia Awareness Day Facts and Stats by Thomas M. Heffron, Mar 10, 2014.
http://www.sleepeducation.org/news/2014/03/10/insomnia-awareness-day-facts-and-stats

10. What is Insomnia? Identifying Sleep Problems.
https://www.insomnia.net/insomnia-faqs/facts/

11. Stress Leads To Lost Sleep, Sedca Ceutics LLC, Overland Park, KS-66207, USA.
http://sedca-ceutics.com/articles/stress-leads-to-lost-sleep.html

12. Journal Publication: Chronic Insomnia Is Associated with Nyctohemeral Activation of the Hypothalamic-Pituitary-Adrenal Axis: Clinical Implications,
J Clin Endocrinol Metab (2001) 86 (8): 3787-3794.
https://academic.oup.com/jcem/article-lookup/doi/10.1210/jcem.86.8.7778

13. Review Posted by Dr. Paul Spector, M.D.
Why You Can't Sleep Through the Night, Nov 21, 2012.
http://www.huffingtonpost.com/paul-spector-md/why-you-might-have-troubl_b_1883811.html

14. Insomnia Statistics, Posted by Better Sleep Better Life, National Sleep Foundation.
http://www.better-sleep-better-life.com/insomnia-statistics.html

15. Insomnia Statistics, Posted by Sleep Cottage, Jan 4, 2010.
http://sleepcottage.com/insomnia-statistics/

16. Sleep & Sleep Disorder Statistics, American Sleep Association, Litiz, PA-17543, USA.
https://www.sleepassociation.org/sleep/sleep-statistics/

17. Sleeping Disorder Statistics, Statistic Brain, Statistic Brain Research Institute, CA-92780, USA.
http://www.statisticbrain.com/sleeping-disorder-statistics/

18. Statistics Posted by Warwick University, Coventry, CV4 7AL, UK.
http://www2.warwick.ac.uk/newsandevents/pressreleases/global_145sleeplessness_epidemic146/

19. INSOMNIA STATISTICS, Posted by Statistics Canada.
http://www.statcan.gc.ca/daily-quotidien/051116/dq051116a-eng.htm

20. INSOMNIA STATISTICS CANADA, Posted bby Michael Tjepkema, Statistics Canada.
http://www.statcan.gc.ca/pub/82-003-x/2005001/article/8707-eng.pdf

21. Insomnia Statistics in Canada: Lack of sleep called 'global epidemic', Doctors press for more shut-eye on World Sleep Day, Posted by CBC News Health, Mar 18, 2011.
http://www.cbc.ca/news/health/lack-of-sleep-called-global-epidemic-1.991855

22. Insomnia & Insomnia Statistics, Posted by Lundbeck (Beijing) Pharmaceutical Consulting Co, Ltd.
http://www.lundbeck.com/cn/en/our-focus/disease-area/insomnia

23. INSOMNIA STATISTICS: A List of 16 Eye-Opening Stats/Facts, by Candace Osmond at Sleep Judge.
https://www.thesleepjudge.com/list-of-insomnia-statistics/

24. 7 Starnge Facts About Insomnia by Linda Thrasybule, MyHealthNewsDaily Contributor, November 30, 2012.
http://www.livescience.com/36454-strange-insomnia-facts-treatments.html

25. Insomnia Statistics by Country, Posted by RightDiagnosis.com.
http://www.rightdiagnosis.com/i/insomnia/stats-country.htm

26. Epidemiology of insomnia: A review of the Global and Indian scenario,
by D Bhattacharya, Manas KAMAL Sen and J C Suri, Vardhman Mahavir Medical College and Safdarjung Hospital, Article (PDF Available), Journal Publication, January 2013.
https://www.researchgate.net/publication/303624977_Epidemiology_of_insomnia_A_review_of_the_Global_and_Indian_scenario

27. Prevalence of insomnia among Chinese adults in Hong Kong: a population-based study by WING S. WONG and RICHARD FIELDING, Department of Applied Social Studies, City University of Hong Kong, Kowloon and Health Behavioral Research Group, School of Public Health, Li Ka Shing Faculty of Medicine, University of Hong Kong, Pokfulam, Hong Kong. Accepted in revised form 04 November 2009; received 20 February 2009.
http://onlinelibrary.wiley.com/doi/10.1111/j.1365-2869.2010.00822.x/pdf

28. Epidemiology of Insomnia, Prevalence and Risk Factors by Claudia de Souza Lopes, Jaqueline Rodrigues Robaina and Lúcia Rotenberg, Institute of Social Medicine, State University of Rio de Janeiro, Brazil (IMS-UERJ), Oswaldo Cruz Institute, Oswaldo Cruz Foundation (IOC-FIOCRUZ).
http://cdn.intechopen.com/pdfs/32269.pdf

29. Prevalence of Insomnia in Europe: A Comparison of 6 Countries.
https://www.ispor.org/research_pdfs/31/pdffiles/PND1.pdf

CHAPTER 3: INSOMNIA SYMPTOMS, CAUSES & RISKS

TABLE OF CONTENTS

WHAT IS INSOMNIA?

Insomnia, also known as sleeplessness, is a sleep disorder because of which people have trouble sleeping, wake up too many times, and spend most of the night tossing and turning on the bed attempting to fall asleep. Usually chronic insomnia sufferers have difficulty falling asleep and maintaining the sleep throughout the night for a prolonged period of time. People who suffer from insomnia are called "insomniacs" or insomnia sufferers.

TYPES OF INSOMNIA [1,2]

a. ACCUTE INSOMNIA (SHORT-TERM INSOMNIA)

Most people go through the acute insomnia problem at some point in their lives, for a period of less than a month, due to temporary stress caused by job loss, preoccupation of keeping the job, noise from neighbors, some kind of illness with pain, long travel, or hormone fluctuations.

b. CHRONIC INSOMNIA (LONG-TERM INSOMNIA)

People who experience insomnia continuously over an extended period of time for more than a month (3 months or more) are considered to be suffering from chronic insomnia and should seek medical advice. People with high levels of stress hormones (more specifically cortisol and adrenocorticotropic hormone (ACTH) or shifts in the levels of cytokines are more likely to suffer from chronic insomnia. Chronic insomnia could develop muscular weariness, fatigue, hallucinations and double vision.

Table 3.1 Difference between acute insomnia and chronic insomnia.

ACUTE INSOMNIA	CHRONIC INSOMNIA
A brief episode of difficulty sleeping. Acute insomnia is usually caused by a life event, such as a stressful change in a person's job, receiving bad news or travel. Acute insomnia can often be treated without any treatment but just by waiting to get back to normal sleep.	A long-term pattern of difficulty sleeping. Chronic insomnia occurs when a person has difficulty sleeping (either falling asleep or maintaining sleep) for at least 3 nights per week for longer than three consecutive months. People with chronic insomnia usually have a long-standing history of difficulty sleeping.

c. LEARNED INSOMNIA & PRIMARY INSOMNIA [3]

Insomnia may even result from a person convincing themselves that they will not be able to sleep, and it is then called "Learned Insomnia". If you believe you have insomnia, then you will have it. That is called "Learned Insomnia". In certain cases, however, there will be no obvious cause to live with insomnia, and this is known as "Primary Insomnia".

d. ONSET INSOMNIA, MIDDLE INSOMNIA, TERMINAL INSOMNIA & HYPERSOMNIA [3a]

If it is taking too long to fall asleep (more than 30 minutes), the person is said to be experiencing initial insomnia or onset insomnia. If the person is waking up too many times and not able to maintain sleep throughout the night, he/she is said to be experiencing interruption insomnia, sleep maintenance insomnia or middle insomnia. If the person wakes up too early in the morning and unable to get back to sleep, he/she is said to be experiencing terminal insomnia. This symptom is primarily associated with depression. Hypersomnia develops if the person is experiencing excessive daytime sleepiness due to sleep apnea, substance abuse or other medical conditions.

INSOMNIA SYMPTOMS & SIGNS [4, 5]

1. You have difficulty falling asleep at night.
2. You wake up frequently during the night and can't go back to sleep.
3. You often feel excessively sleepy throughout the day after you wake up.
4. You frequently experience fatigue and are moody, irritable, cranky or over-emotional.
5. You struggle to stay alert while driving, or during meetings/movies, etc.
6. You often feel anxious and even depressed.
7. Caffeine drinks, smoking (nicotine) and alcohol are a normal part of your life.
8. One or some of the medications are probably exhibiting their side effects.
9. You are suffering from other medical conditions that you are not aware of.
10. You feel tired and dissatisfied even after a good night's sleep.
11. Your partner says you snore loudly and are disturbing other sleepers.

Insomnia symptoms extend beyond a pattern of sleeplessness, negatively affecting the wellness the normal energy levels, if left untreated: [6]

12. **Mood Swings:** If you find yourself easily upset, agitated, angry, frustrated or feel like you are on an emotional roller coaster, it means you are not getting sufficient sleep during the night (check yourself!).

13. **Poor Coordination:** If you find yourself becoming clumsy, have trouble paying attention to simple tasks, drop things frequently on the floor, stumble when walking by losing consciousness instantly, your hands bump into objects, and you are unable to complete scheduled tasks as planned, check yourself. You could be suffering from insomnia, and treatment is necessary. Insomnia has repercussions. It impacts your work/school life by resulting in poor productivity.

14. **Memory Problems:** If you are becoming forgetful, don't remember names, dates and incidents that are necessary in your daily life, lose items and don't remember where you placed or hid them and feel mentally blank, it indicates that your brain is unable to store and organize memories properly and is preventing recollection. Here again, insomnia is to be blamed. You need to cleanse your brain through sufficient sleep.

15. **Anxiety & Depression:** Sleep deprivation or chronic insomnia can lead to even more dangerous health conditions and health disorders such as anxiety and depression, as the chemical balance of your brain is disrupted by poor sleep patterns. Further, anxiety and depression could act against and further complicate your sleep–wake cycle. Your master biological clock is disturbed and is no longer under your brain's control. You should take action.

16. **Poor Physical Condition:** Over time, insomniacs could develop physical problems such as ongoing headaches, high blood pressure, weight gain and falling asleep on the wheel while driving, totally out of control. Immediate action is required to treat your chronic insomnia.

INSOMNIA CAUSES [3, 5, 6, 7, 8]

CAUSES OF ACUTE INSOMNIA
♦ Many factors can cause insomnia. Stress, anxiety and depression are common causes. Caffeine, nicotine and alcohol, and many prescription drugs that have side effects can also interfere with the sleep, and could cause sleeplessness.
♦ Breathing disorder due to nasal blockage and airway in the throat blockage could cause insomnia.
♦ Females are twice as likely to suffer from acute insomnia than men.
♦ A shift in hormone levels for women during the period of menstruation and menopause is associated with the disruption in sleep patterns. A shift in the hormone levels of serotonin, progesterone and estrogen can be accompanied by night sweats, hot flashes, vivid dreams and nightmares. This kind of activity could trigger a biochemical stress and turn into the emotional stress, causing sleeplessness during the night.
♦ Seniors, people over 65, are more likely to suffer from acute insomnia than people under 65-years old. REM sleep is expected to decrease with age.
♦ Indigestion, constipation and heart disease, if left untreated, could cause acute insomnia.
♦ Psychological causes such as anxiety and depression can cause acute insomnia.
♦ Illnesses, including mental illness, surgery, or injuries that cause a period of pain and discomfort can lead to acute insomnia.
♦ Shift work late at night could shift your master biological clock, and lead to acute insomnia.
♦ Jet-Lag (frequent travels by taking flights to different time zones) could disrupt the circadian rhythm, and could change the sleep-wake cycle. Eventually it could lead to acute insomnia.
♦ Some junk foods, street drugs, too much alcohol consumption, smoking (nicotine), caffeine drinks, and some medications could cause acute insomnia.

CAUSES OF CHRONIC INSOMNIA
♦ Acute insomnia over time could turn into the primary cause of chronic insomnia.
♦ Chronic health conditions such as arthritis, asthma, heart problems, acid reflux disease, restless legs syndrome, fibromyalgia, high blood pressure, tinnitus (ringing in the ears), as well as diseases such as alzheimers and parkinsons could make a person feel discomfort and overly stressful throughout the night, and could lead to chronic insomnia.
♦ Chronic pain related to the aforementioned health conditions (especially fibromyalgia) could keep you awake all the night, causing chronic insomnia.
♦ Sleep apnea suffers could also suffer from insomnia. Whenever a person stops breathing for more than 10 seconds (whenever the apnea comes in), the person is awakened by the brain in order to breathe. Too many apneas means, too many awakenings by the brain. This kind of activity due to sleep apnea causes insomnia.
♦ Genetics and heredity could play a role. If a person in the family suffered from chronic insomnia, that person could be at risk of developing the same sleep disorder (insomnia).

INSOMNIA RISKS AND COMPLICATIONS

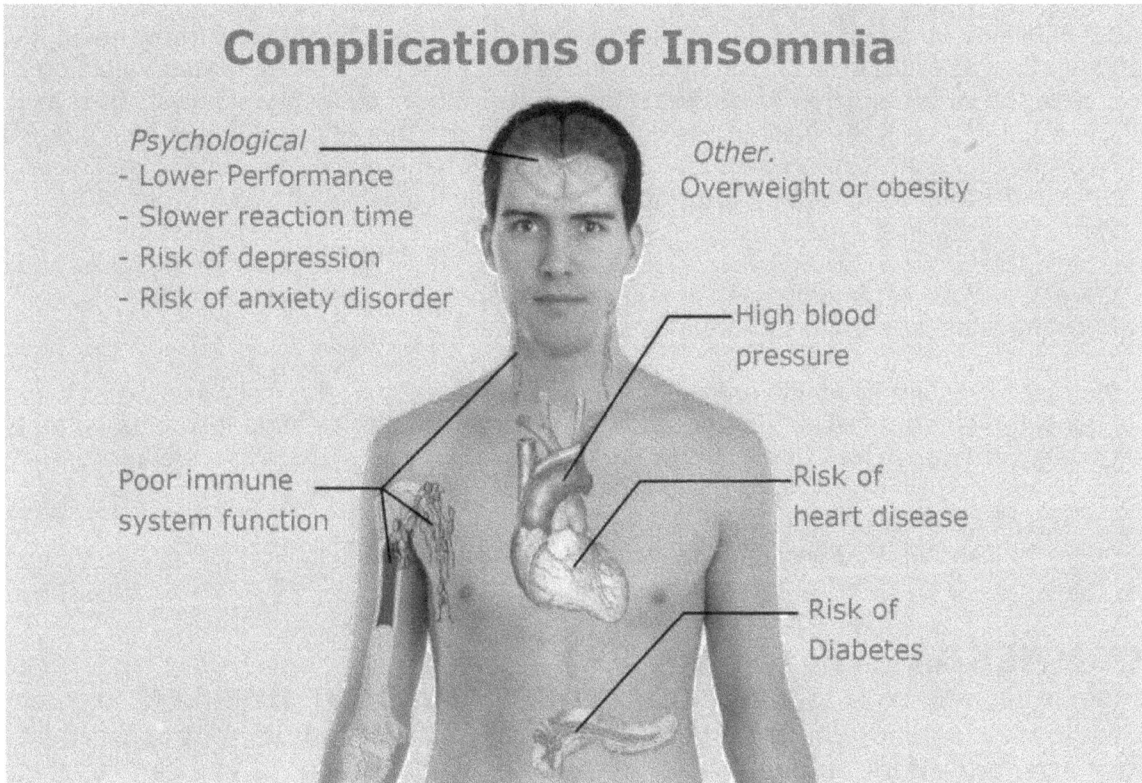

Figure 3.1 Complications of insomnia.

SLEEP DEPRIVATION [9, 10]

Deprivation means the state of not having something that people need or people lost. When you do not enjoy sufficient sleep at night indefinitely for extended periods of time, you lost your sleep, and you most likely are suffering from sleep deprivation, chronic insomnia, interrupted sleep or impaired sleep. Sleep deprivation is dangerous to your health and could develop any of the following health conditions and/or health disorders.

- ◆ Poor sleep lowers performance and makes your life miserable in every possible way.
- ◆ It increases stress and could dramatically weaken your immune system.
- ◆ It could cause severe yawning.
- ◆ It could cause cognitive (mental process of perception) impairment.
- ◆ It could lead you to pre-diabetic state, making you feel hungry and eat more, and gain weight.
- ◆ It could cause stress-related disorders such as a heart disease, high blood pressure, increased heart rate, stomach ulcers, constipation, mood disorders, anxiety disorder, memory loss and even depression.
- ◆ It could quickly increase tumor growth.
- ◆ It could ultimately lead to death.

LIGHT THERAPY FOR INSOMNIA [11]

Light therapy is used to cure insomnia. In light therapy, the insomnia patient is exposed to a special light box for a certain amount of time each day. The artificial light from the light-therapy box mimics outdoor sunlight (from sunrise to sunset) so that the patient's biological clock and so the circadian rhythm is reset. More specifically, the sleep-wake cycle of the patient is regulated until the insomnia is wiped out. In light therapy, the unit is designed so that the ultraviolet light is filtered and it would be safe for the eyes. The patient is allowed to read, sit in front of a computer, write or do other activities while sitting in front of the light box.

Light therapy is most commonly used in countries where is sun does not come out so often and where the sunlight is hard to find in the environment.

Light therapy boxes are available online. It is always advised that the insomnia patient should consult his/her physician or sleep specialist who has been treating insomnia patients using the light therapy. Light therapy could adversely affect the eyesight so the appropriate precautions are to be taken while using the light box.

Please refer to Chapter 1 where light therapy treatment is explained.

RECOMMENDATION (by Dr. RK)

This course recommends that you "**DO NOT USE ANY LIGHT THERAPY**" to treat your insomnia. Instead, you treat your insomnia naturally from its root cause by following the procedure outlined in 24 instructions in Chapter 1. If you can reset your suprachiasmatic nucleus (SCN) or master biological clock, your sleep-wake cycle will automatically be restored, and then you will be able to sleep like a baby. You can do that in less than a week by properly exposing yourself to darkness at night. Your brain is capable of naturally secreting as much melatonin as the body needs during the night, from the pineal gland. Melatonin is essential to fall asleep and remain asleep throughout the night, and to restore the normal sleep-wake cycle. Please read Chapter 1 of this book, and follow the step-by-step instructions (24 instructions) outlined to treat your insomnia.

SLEEPING PILLS ARE DANGEROUS

SLEEPING PILLS ARE HARMFUL TO YOUR HEALTH
♦ Sleeping pills are hazardous to your health and could cause death from cancer, heart disease, or other illnesses. This means that people who take sleeping pills die sooner than people who do not use sleeping pills. [12]

♦ Patients who took sleeping pills died 4.6 times more often (on an average) than patients who avoided sleeping pills. If sleeping pills cause even a small portion of the excess deaths and cancers associated with their use, they are too dangerous to use. [12]

♦ There is documented evidence that sleeping pills cause cancer. [12]

♦ Sleeping pills, if consumed prolonged time, could damage the liver.

AMBIEN WAS FOUND TO BE THE MOST DANGEROUS SLEEPING PILL
♦ Ambien was found to be the most dangerous sleeping pill. The side effects of Ambien are drowsiness during the day, dizziness, sleepiness and drowsiness when driving, sleep-walking and hallucinations. Many people experienced these side effects and caused automobile accidents while sleep-driving, and their entire lives have been ruined after taking the sleeping pill "AMBIEN". [13, 14]

♦ Dr. Anthony Komaroff (Dr. K) and his colleague Dr. Suzanne Salamon of Harvard Medical School recommend that it not safe to take a sleeping pill every night, especially if you are a senior (over 65). [15] They also recommend the book of Dr. Lawrence Epstein and Dr. Steven Mardon titled "The Harvard Medical School Guide to a Good Night's Sleep." [16] They suggested that it is always better to resolve the insomnia problem from its root cause rather than depending on sleeping pills.

♦ Sleeping pills are addictive. You may have to increase the dosage every now and then for it to be effective, a habit that leads to daytime grogginess and may contribute to cognitive problems (mental perception is retarded), poor balance and could even lead to falling asleep on the wheel while driving.

LIST OF SLEEPING PILLS AND DRUG THERAPY [17, 18, 19]

The following prescription drugs help fall asleep:
    a. Eszopiclone (Lunesta)
    b. Ramelteon (Rozerem)
    c. Triazolam (Halcion)
    d. Zaleplon (Sonata)
    e. Zolpidem (Ambien)

The following prescription drugs help maintain sleep:
    a. Estazolam
    b. Eszopiclone (Lunesta)
    c. Temazepam (Restoril)
    d. Zolpidem (Ambien CR)

The following prescription drugs are used for insomnia and depression:
    a. Amitriptyline
    b. Nortriptyline (Pamelor)
    c. Trazodone (Desyrel)
    d. Eszopiclone (Oral Route)
    e. Ramelteon (Oral Route)
    f. Zaleplon (Oral Route)
    g. Zolpidem (Oral Route, Oromucosal Route)
    h. Trazodone (Oral Route)

There are many sleep-aids and non-prescription drugs available over the counter without prescription. The most well-known pills are melatonin, unisom and valerian root. Melatonin is the most famous pill and it could help some people to fall asleep at the beginning of the night for some time. After some time, after prolonged usage, it may not work.

ARTIFICIAL MELATONIN
Some people take artificial melatonin to improve their sleep disorder but it is not guaranteed to work. It works for some people for some time, and may not work for others for all the times they take it. Sometimes it looks like it is working, but after taking it continuously, it stops working as expected. It is up to the individual to research by trying all possible ways to find out if melatonin is beneficial or not and if it induces sleep or not when needed.

Melatonin: Melatonin is a natural hormone produced by the pineal gland located in your brain. When the natural melatonin production depletes due to a sleep disorder, you can supplement it by taking artificial melatonin found over the counter without any prescription. It is suggested to take this artificial melatonin starting from a low dose and then gradually increase the dosage day after day until you find the appropriate dosage that suits you and makes you sleepy. Also follow the dosage instructions printed on the label. Melatonin liquid drops work more effectively than the tablets.

RECOMMENDATION (by Dr. RK)
This course recommends that you "**DO NOT USE ANY PRESCRIPTION SLEEPING PILLS**" to treat your insomnia. Instead, you better treat your insomnia naturally from its root-cause by following the procedure outlined in this course. Go to the MAIN ARTICLE of this course and follow all the 24 step-by-step instructions outlined in this course to treat your insomnia. If you can reset your suprachiasmatic nucleus (SCN) or master biological clock, your sleep-wake cycle will automatically be restored, and then you will be able to sleep like a baby. You can do that in less than a week by properly exposing to sunshine or bright lights during the day, and by living in the dark at night. Your brain is capable of naturally secreting as much melatonin as the body needs during the night, from the pineal gland. Melatonin is essential to fall asleep and remain asleep throughout the night, and to restore the normal sleep-wake cycle. Artificial melatonin is unnecessary and, after a certain time, it won't work as it is supposed to be working.

REFERENCES

1. Insomnia (from Wikipedia).
https://en.wikipedia.org/wiki/Insomnia

2. Insomnia Causes and Cures: What to Do When You Cannot Sleep?
https://www.helpguide.org/articles/sleep/cant-sleep-insomnia-treatment.htm

3. Insomnia & Insomnia Statistics, Posted by Lundbeck (Beijing) Pharmaceutical Consulting Co, Ltd.
http://www.lundbeck.com/cn/en/our-focus/disease-area/insomnia

3a. Sleep Disorders Clinical Presentation, Author: Roy H Lubit, MD, PhD; Chief Editor: Iqbal Ahmed, MBBS, FRCPsych(UK), Updated: Jan 28, 2015.
https://emedicine.medscape.com/article/287104-clinical

4. Insomnia Test, The Better Sleep Guide, Better Sleep Better Life.
http://www.better-sleep-better-life.com/insomnia-test.html

5. 10 Signs of Insomnia, Posted by Kimberly Love, April 18, 2016.
http://rmhealthy.com/10-signs-insomnia/

6. 10 Causes of Insomnia by Dorathy Gass, February 22, 2015.
http://rmhealthy.com/10-causes-insomnia/

7. Recognizing Insomnia Symptoms, Better Sleep Better Life.
http://www.better-sleep-better-life.com/insomnia-symptoms.html

8. Causes of Insomnia, The Better Sleep Guide, Better Sleep Better Life.
http://www.better-sleep-better-life.com/causes-of-insomnia.html

9. Stress Leads to Lost Sleep, Sedca Ceutics LLC, Overland Park, KS-66207, USA.
http://sedca-ceutics.com/articles/stress-leads-to-lost-sleep.html

10. Journal Publication: Chronic Insomnia Is Associated with Nyctohemeral Activation of the Hypothalamic-Pituitary-Adrenal Axis: Clinical Implications,
J Clin Endocrinol Metab (2001) 86 (8): 3787-3794.
https://academic.oup.com/jcem/article-lookup/doi/10.1210/jcem.86.8.7778

11. Light Therapy for Insomnia Sufferers.
https://sleepfoundation.org/insomnia/content/light-therapy-insomnia-sufferers

12. The Dark Side of Sleeping Pills by Daniel F. Kripke, MD.
http://www.darksideofsleepingpills.com/

13. Why Ambien and Other Sleeping Aids Are Very Dangerous and May Need to Be Off the Market; Despite the hazardous side effects, there is a huge market for insomnia drugs.
http://www.alternet.org/drugs/why-ambien-and-other-sleeping-aids-are-very-dangerous-and-may-need-be-market

14. Danger of Ambien.
https://www.healthstatus.com/health_blog/sleep-2/danger-ambien/

15. Is It Safe to Take Sleeping Pill Every Night?
by Dr. Anthony Komaroff, Harvard Medical School, April 18, 2012.
http://www.askdoctork.com/is-it-safe-to-take-a-sleeping-pill-every-night-201204181656

16. The Harvard Medical School Guide to a Good Night's Sleep Paperback
by Dr. Lawrence Epstein and Dr. Steven Mardon, Oct 16 2006.
https://www.amazon.ca/Harvard-Medical-School-Guide-Nights/dp/0071467432

17. List of Sleeping Pills by Sharon Durmaskin, eHow Contributor.
http://www.ehow.com/facts_5315329_list-sleeping-pills.html

18. Comparison of Sleeping Pills: Which is The Best and The Worst?
http://www.emedexpert.com/compare/sleeping-pills.shtml

19. Insomnia Drugs and Dosages, Drug Therapy, Sleep Disorders by Cleveland Clinic.
http://www.clevelandclinicmeded.com/medicalpubs/diseasemanagement/neurology/sleep-disorders/

CHAPTER 4: MIDDLE-OF-THE-NIGHT INSOMNIA IS A NORMAL SLEEP PATTERN

TABLE OF CONTENTS

Dr. THOMAS WEHR'S RESEARCH STUDY [1, 2]
Middle-of-the-Night Insomnia Could Be A Normal Sleep Pattern

The American psychiatrist Dr. Thomas Alvin Wehr received his degree in medicine from the University of Louisville School of Medicine in 1969. He subsequently completed his psychiatric residency at Yale School of Medicine and his internship was at Michael Reese Hospital. Dr. Wehr was a Scientist Emeritus at the National Institute of Mental Health (NIMH), and former chief of the Clinical Psychobiology branch at NIMH.

During 1990s, the American psychiatrist Dr. Thomas Wehr conducted a study on photoperiodicity in humans to understand the sleep-wake cycle. He selected 8 healthy sleepers (8 healthy men) who were not troubled with insomnia at that time and who were accustomed to live in 16 to 17 hours of daytime and 8 or 7 hours of nighttime for sleep. He placed them in a strictly organized quiet room so that the bright lights would be turned on during the daytime hours and turned off during the nighttime hours in order to expose them to dark every night. All the 8 subjects were hooked up with sticky patches and sensors/electrodes on their scalp, face, chest, limbs and a finger, and were asked to sleep as long as they could so that the lab technician could monitor exactly how many hours they slept and how many hours they remained awake. Their melatonin levels were also supposed to be monitored during the night.

He then exposed them to 10 hours of bright light per day (creating the daytime) and 14 hours of dark per day (creating the nighttime) and watched, and monitored everything that happened during their sleep. This ratio of light to dark (10:14) mimics the natural weather of a typical winter day in a temperate climate region. Initially, they slept for 11 hours per night, suggesting chronic sleep deficit or chronic sleep debt, and then settled into an average of 8.9 hours each night. By the fourth week, Dr. Wehr inadvertently stumbled on something that changed everything about sleep-wake cycle of humans. All 8 sleepers developed a sleep pattern characterized by two sleep sessions in two phases or two segments: All 8 subjects, when they were exposed to dark, tended to lie awake for 1 to 2 hours, and then fall quickly asleep. After about 4 hours of solid sleep, they would remain awake and spend 1 to 2 hours in a state of quiet wakefulness, experiencing some sort of INSOMNIA, and then they slept for another 4 hours. Which means they slept in two segments: 4 hours in the first segment and another 4 hours in the second segment. Dr. Wehr also observed that there was a spike in their melatonin levels during the phase-II sleep or second segment.

CONCLUSIONS
(i) Dr. Thomas Wehr interpreted that such a biphasic sleep-wake pattern (4 hours of sleep in phase-I, stay awake for 2 to 3 hours, and sleep another 4 hours in phase-II) was natural and agrees with the pre-historic sleep tendency for humans in ancient times before electricity was discovered. Our ancestors, several hundred years ago, before the towns, cities, houses and offices were illuminated by electricity, used to live in the dark at night, and they rarely suffered from chronic insomnia. At that time, the sleep pattern in humans was biphasic.

(ii) As the darkness intensified late at night, the retinas sensed more and more darkness and sent signals to the Suprachiasmatic Nucleus (SCN) or the master biological clock, embedded in the hypothalamus of the brain, which ordered the pineal gland to produce more melatonin. That was the reason why there was a spike in melatonin level during the phase-II sleep.

(iii) Dr. Thomas Wehr also interpreted that that long sleep of 11 hours, during the first week, was due to the repaying of chronic sleep debt or sleep deficit those subjects accumulated as they probably did not sleep enough (at least 8 hours per day) in the near past so their brains demanded more sleep when they were exposed to darkness for 14 hours per night.

(iv) In the later stages of his investigation, Dr. Thomas Wehr and his fellow-researchers concluded that the brain produces high levels of the pituitary hormone called "prolactin" during the period of nighttime wakefulness (during the period of middle-of-the-night-insomnia), which may contribute to the feeling of peace and happiness during the day. Which means the middle-of-the-night insomnia is good for you.

Meaning of Photoperiod = The daily duration of light and dark to which an organism is exposed, considered especially with regard to its effect on growth and development; The period of daylight in every 24 hours, especially in relation to its effects on plants and animals; The interval in a 24-hour period during which a plant or animal is exposed to light.

Segmented Sleep

Segmented sleep also known as divided sleep or interrupted sleep, is a sleep pattern where two or more periods of sleep are punctuated by a period of wakefulness. Along with a nap/siesta in the day, it has been argued that this in fact is the natural pattern of human sleep and helps to regulate stress.

Figure 4.1 Dr. Thomas Wehr's research summary.

DR. ROGER EKIRCH'S WORK ON SEGMENTED SLEEP [3]

Historian Dr. Roger Ekirch was a professor of History in Virginia Tech. He has argued that before the Industrial Revolution, segmented sleep was the dominant form of human sleep in the Western civilization. He draws evidence from documents of the ancient, medieval, and modern world.

Dr. Roger Ekirch collected a lot of ancient information about how the people used to sleep from personal diaries, medical records, court documents, etc., and published a 500-page book in 2005 entitled "At Day's Close: Night in Times Past". [3]

This book revels that segmented sleep is normal. Sleeping for 3 hours, lying awake for 2 to 3 hours and sleeping again till morning. In the ancient times, people used to sleep like that. People get up in the middle of the night, read a book, talk to each other, couples make sex, or even go out and talk to neighbors, etc. Then go back to bed and sleep till morning.

Segmented sleep, also known as divided sleep, bimodal sleep pattern, bifurcated sleep, or interrupted sleep, is a polyphasic sleep or biphasic sleep pattern where two or more periods of sleep are punctuated by periods of wakefulness. Along with a nap (siesta) in the day, it has been argued that this is the natural pattern of human sleep. A case has been made that maintaining such a sleep pattern may be important in regulating stress.

As A Historical Norm [4]

According to Professor Dr. Roger Ekirch's argument, typically individuals slept in two distinct phases bridged by an intervening period of wakefulness of approximately 1 to 2 hours. Some people used to pray in groups and interpret dreams. Some scholars took advantage of fruitful thoughts and used to write both poetry and prose. Whereas some others visited neighbors, engaged in sex, or committed petty crime.

The brain produces high levels of the pituitary hormone called "prolactin" during the period of nighttime wakefulness, which may contribute to the feeling of peace and happiness.

The two distinct phases of sleep at night, according to Ekirch's theory, were first sleep (also called dead sleep) and second sleep (also called morning sleep). Different people used different names in different languages by translating the first sleep and second sleep.

The circadian rhythm regulates the human sleep-wake cycle, by staying awake during the day and by sleeping at night. Dr. Roger Ekirch suggested that due to the modern era of electric lighting, people stopped practicing segmented sleep.

Research on sleep patterns

Dr.Ekirch's research makes the claim that normally, humans didn't always sleep for about 8 hours all at once. Instead, he found that humans appear to have slept in two shorter periods at night beginning with 3 or 4 hours of sleep and then followed by being awake for 3 hours or so, then sleeping again until daybreak.

All of this occured within a 12-hour time frame

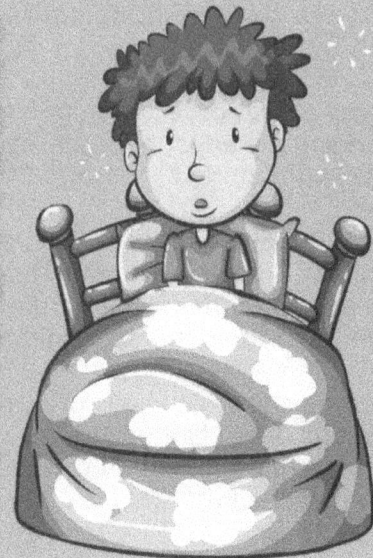

Figure 4.2 Dr. Roger Ekirch's research summary.

Review Posted by Susannah Ottaway [5]

Ekirch argues that before the introduction of artificial light, people's sleep was actually broken into two parts: "first sleep", followed by a period of an hour or so when individuals experienced restful meditation ("quiet wakefulness", p. 300), and then a second sleep through to morning time. Ekirch concludes that pre-industrial sleep patterns were profoundly different from our own, and that the opportunity to lie awake and reflect on their dreams in the middle of the night "allowed many to absorb fresh visions before returning to unconsciousness," visions that may have been "sources of self-revelation, solace and spirituality" (322). While this is a fascinating idea that may offer profound insights into early modern psyches, more direct evidence and deeper analysis of this phenomenon is necessary to render this conclusion completely compelling.

Review Posted by Ian Pindar [6]

The book's most fascinating revelation is that our pre-industrial ancestors experienced what Dr. Roger Ekirch calls "segmented sleep": there was "first sleep" until midnight, then a "second sleep". In between, they tended the fire, read or talked, had sex, smoked and meditated on the events of the previous day. Electric lighting has altered our sleep patterns and robbed us of this nocturnal hiatus.

In fact, Ekirch contends that the "gradual elimination" of night has actually impaired the quality of our dreams and deprived us of "a better understanding of our inner selves". What began as a history of nighttime becomes by the end a lament for a night we have lost.

DR. CRAIG KOFLOFSKY'S WORK ON SEGMENTED SLEEP [7, 8]

Other historians, such as Dr. Craig Koflofsky (Professor of History, Germanic Languages and Literatures, University of Illinois at Chicago) have endorsed Dr. Roger Ekirch's analysis on segmented sleep.

Dr. Craig Koflofsky published the following book in 2011. [8]
Dr. Craig Koflofsky's Book: Evening's Empire: A History of the Night in Early Modern Europe, Cambridge University Press, 2011.

What does it mean to write a history of the night? Evening's Empire is a fascinating study of the myriad ways in which early modern people understood, experienced and transformed the night. Using diaries, letters, and legal records together with representations of the night in early modern religion, literature and art, Dr. Craig Koflofsky opens up an entirely new perspective on early modern Europe. He shows how princes, courtiers, burghers and common people 'nocturnalized' political expression, the public sphere and the use of daily time. Fear of the night was now mingled with improved opportunities for labour and leisure: the modern night was beginning to assume its characteristic shape. Evening's Empire takes the evocative history of the night into early modern politics, culture and society, revealing its importance to key themes from witchcraft, piety, and gender to colonization, race and the Enlightenment.

Review Posted by Prof. Joad Raymond [9]
Published in History Today Volume 62 Issue 2 February 2012
Joad Raymond is a Professor of English Literature at the University of East Anglia.

This engaging book, the winner of the Longman-History Today Prize for 2011, examines the practices and cultural meanings attached to something both ubiquitous and (at least historiographically) almost invisible: the night and its attendant darkness. It proposes that in 16th and 17th century Europe, the boundaries of night were driven back and simultaneously the associations of darkness were enriched and transformed. The schedule of the day changed. The traditional two-part, segmented sleep (with a waking interval) of rural communities was replaced in cities with a single phase of sleep. The schedule of the urban day slipped back, so rising, mealtimes and sleep occurred later. But the meaning of the night also changed – its symbolisms and associations were re-imagined and re-invented.

Evening's Empire offers a fertile and richly European account of deep and sometimes unexpected cultural associations, exploring witchcraft, religion, court spectacle, street lighting, coffee houses, the urban-rural divide and enlightenment.

Dr. Koslofsky's night is both real and imaginary. The process of 'nocturnalisation' he describes, involves the invasion of the hours of darkness, the associated dispelling of darkness and a cultural shift – a 'revolution' he suggests – manifested in several contrasting domains. By the late 16th century, darkness was no longer simply negative, the province of demons and witches. Instead it became also a time for spiritual insight, for comprehending the ineffable Word. This was especially so for those Protestant sects that were obliged, through persecution, to worship under cover of night. Yet it was not only radical Protestants who reinvested night with spiritual revelation. The figure of Nicodemus suggested to wider networks of Christians the nocturnal arrival of spiritual light.

However, the weakening of the traditional association of darkness with malign spirits was uneven. While scholars (using the dichotomies characteristic of European intellectual culture at this time) pushed to associate the night with diabolical activity, popular culture preserved a view in which some nocturnal activities – such as spinning bees, night-time meetings, where women's labour sometimes served as a pretence for courtship – were regarded as intrinsically ambivalent or positive.

There was a practical dimension to these developments. The night retreated under the glare of street lighting, which transformed urban spaces and enabled new uses for streets at night. Across Europe it was variously imposed by princes or voluntarily introduced by city governors. By contrast stage lighting meant that European courts exploited darkness as a context for theatrical spectacles that magnified the glory of the ruler. Nocturnal theatre invaded night's territories and used the dark for cultural, civilized purposes. While light was associated with power and virtue only, through its relationship with darkness was this association maintained and by this means the reciprocity of the two was recognized, much as in chiaroscuro painting.

Another nocturnal cultural activity involved coffee houses. Dr. Koslofsky argues that debates usually took place during evening, another sign of the advance of culture into later hours. The urban night ceased to be a time fraught with danger, outlaws and vice and became a socially acceptable occasion for cultural activity. The night became polite. However, like the public sphere of popular opinion itself, this shift was not gender blind – nocturnal activity by women continued to be morally suspected.

With politeness came two means by which nocturnalisation was associated with enlightenment. The Enlightenment involved conversations that took place at night and its written texts picked up on the light-dark dichotomy to articulate Europe's self-proclaimed superiority over the unenlightened or pagan world. The central trope of the Enlightenment, therefore, was invested in this process of nocturnalisation. This philosophical use of night was in some respects reductive: while in many other contexts the night was placed on both sides of a series of antitheses, Enlightenment philosophers positioned it as simply negative. This incomplete summary indicates the richness of the book. My criticisms are minor: there is no discussion of latitude (or longitude) and some of Dr. Koslofsky's themes are supported by insufficient evidence – the use of darkness in court poetry or in the language of the stage, for example – which in any case only indirectly relate to the process of nocturnalisation and do not contribute to his chronology. However, a fully schematic version would undoubtedly misrepresent the shaded contours of reality. Instead Dr. Koslofsky offers a rich series of sketches from incomplete perspectives that suggest the intensive associations of night and a broad pattern of change. This is a valuable contribution to the history of the everyday and, especially, of the experience of temporality.

Review Posted by Adam McDowell [10]
Rest assured: There's Nothing Wrong with Segmented Sleep

Segmented sleep: Rest assured there's nothing wrong with waking up a few times during the night.

Bad sleepers rarely hear good news. Insomniacs often read about the latest ways our nighttime pacing is believed to be wrecking our health. Or we are treated to recycled and often unrealistic advice about how to shift around our routines to encourage sounder sleep. We can feel guilty if we find ourselves unable to follow it.

So my curiosity was piqued when a recent BBC online story, "The myth of the eight-hour sleep," shone a light on a growing body of research suggesting that "segmented sleep" is perfectly normal. It appears that in centuries past, and in pre-industrial societies, bedtime has meant falling asleep once, then waking for awhile, and then going back to bed for a "second sleep".

"That sounds like me", I thought — as many others surely did. Historians are arguing that everyone used to spend the night that way. For those who wake up in the middle of the night, this could be liberating news.

Before artificial lighting "colonized" the darkness (borrowing a term from the historian Dr. Craig Koslofsky), a nightly wakeful interlude was expected. Lighting and caffeinated beverages promoted active, chatty evenings. This, historians believe, pushed back the Western world's bedtime. The modern ideal of a continuous eight-hour slumber was born. But prior to that, the idea of a "first" and "second" sleep was so routine, one researcher wrote, "it provoked little comment at the time."

This was the insight of Dr. Roger Ekirch, a professor of history at Virginia Tech. In his 2005 book 'At Day's Close', he argued that: "Until the close of the early modern era [roughly the year 1800], Western Europeans on most evenings experienced two major of sleep segments bridged by an hour or more of quiet wakefulness." This period was known as the "watch" or "watching."

"Segmented sleep has a lot of historical evidence," says Dr. Koslofsky, an associate professor of history at the University of Illinois and author of last fall's 'Evening's Empire: A History of the Night in Early Modern Europe'. "Ekirch really demonstrated that these terms, 'first' and 'second' sleep, appeared in Homer, in Virgil, in ancient medieval Christian literature," he says. Humbler literature including diaries and prayer books also contain clues to how Westerners slept in the past. Segmented sleep, Dr. Koslofsky says, "also seems to appear in societies that don't have a lot of access to artificial light. ... I think it's a natural feature of human evolution to break any long, dark period up into two sleeps."

Take the Trumai, an indigenous people in Brazil. They used to get up in the middle of the night to socialize and flirt by the fireside, smoke, or go fishing. The introduction of electricity to their society put an end to their midnight wanderings. Similar behaviour has been documented in other cultures. If biphasic slumber is common, could it be the "correct" way to sleep? That is, did evolution design us for two four-hour chunks of rest? What is ideal, anyway?

Review Posted by Stephanie Hegarty [11]
The Myth of An Eight-Hour Sleep

We often worry about lying awake in the middle of the night - but it could be good for you. A growing body of evidence from both science and history suggests that the eight-hour sleep may be unnatural.

In the early 1990s, psychiatrist Dr. Thomas Wehr conducted an experiment in which a group of people were plunged into darkness for 14 hours every day for a month. It took some time for their sleep to regulate but by the fourth week, the subjects had settled into a very distinct sleeping pattern. They slept first for four hours, then woke for one or two hours before falling into a second four-hour sleep. Though sleep scientists were impressed by the study, among the general public the idea that we must sleep for eight consecutive hours persists.

In 2001, historian Dr. Roger Ekirch of Virginia Tech published a seminal paper, drawn from 16 years of research, revealing a wealth of historical evidence that humans used to sleep in two distinct chunks. His book 'At Day's Close: Night in Times Past', published four years later, unearths more than 500 references to a segmented sleeping pattern - in diaries, court records, medical books and literature, from Homer's Odyssey to an anthropological account of modern tribes in Nigeria.

Much like the experience of Wehr's subjects, these references describe a first sleep which began about two hours after dusk, followed by waking period of one or two hours and then a second sleep.

During this waking period people were quite active. They often got up, went to the toilet or smoked tobacco and some even visited neighbors. Most people stayed in bed, read, wrote and often prayed. Countless prayer manuals from the late 15th Century offered special prayers for the hours in between sleeps.

And these hours weren't entirely solitary - people often chatted to bed-fellows or had sex. A doctor's manual from 16th Century France even advised couples that the best time to conceive was not at the end of a long day's labour but "after the first sleep", when "they have more enjoyment" and "do it better".

Ekirch found that references to the first and second sleep started to disappear during the late 17th Century. This started among the urban upper classes in northern Europe and over the course of the next 200 years filtered down to the rest of Western society.

By the 1920s the idea of a first and second sleep had receded entirely from our social consciousness.

He attributes the initial shift to improvements in street lighting, domestic lighting and a surge in coffee houses - which were sometimes open all night. As the night became a place for legitimate activity and as that activity increased, the length of time people could dedicate to rest dwindled (become smaller).

In his new book, 'Evening's Empire', historian Dr. Craig Koslofsky puts forward an account of how this happened. "Associations with night before the 17th Century were not good", he says. The night was a place populated by people of disrepute - criminals, prostitutes and drunks. "Even the wealthy, who could afford candlelight, had better things to spend their money on. There was no prestige or social value associated with staying up all night."

That changed in the wake of the Reformation and the counter-Reformation. Protestants and Catholics became accustomed to holding secret services at night, during periods of persecution. If earlier the night had belonged to reprobates, now respectable people became accustomed to exploiting the hours of darkness. This trend migrated to the social sphere too, but only for those who could afford to live by candlelight. With the advent of street lighting, however, socialising at night began to filter down through the classes.

In many historic accounts, Ekirch found that people used the time to meditate on their dreams. "Today we spend less time doing those things", says Dr. Jacobs. "It's not a coincidence that, in modern life, the number of people who report anxiety, stress, depression, alcoholism and drug abuse has gone up". So the next time you wake up in the middle of the night, think of your pre-industrial ancestors and relax. Lying awake could be good for you.

Every 60-100 minutes we go through a cycle of four stages of sleep:
♦ Stage 1 is a drowsy, relaxed state between being awake and sleeping - breathing slows, muscles relax, heart rate drops.
♦ Stage 2 is slightly deeper sleep - you may feel awake and this means that, on many nights, you may be asleep and not know it.
♦ Stage 3 and Stage 4, or Deep Sleep - it is very hard to wake up from Deep Sleep because this is when there is the lowest amount of activity in your body.
♦ After Deep Sleep, we go back to Stage 2 for a few minutes, and then enter Dream Sleep - also called REM (rapid eye movement) sleep - which, as its name suggests, is when you dream.
In a full sleep cycle, a person goes through all the stages of sleep from one to four, then back down through stages three and two, before entering dream sleep.

Review Posted by Dr. Walter A. Brown, MD [12]
Broken Sleep May Be Natural Sleep

Dr. Brown is a clinical professor of psychiatry at Brown Medical School, Providence, RI, and Tufts University School of Medicine, Boston, and a practicing psychiatrist.

Sleep In Times Past: In his book about nights in the Pre-industrial times "At Day's Close: Night in Times Past", Dr. Roger Ekirch, professor of history at Virginia Polytechnic Institute, uncovered the fact that before artificial illumination was widely used, people typically slept in 2 bouts, which they called first sleep and second sleep. In those times, sleep was more closely tied to sunset and sunrise than it is now. Within an hour or so after sunset, people retired to bed, slept for about 4 hours, and then woke up. They remained awake for a couple of hours and then returned to sleep at about 2 am for another 4 hours or so till the sun rises in the morning.

Written records from before the first century onward indicate that the period between first and second sleep offered a chance for quiet contemplation, but people also got out of bed during this interval and did household chores or visited family and friends. Although diaries, court documents, and literature of the time indicate that this sleep pattern was widely known and acknowledged, until Ekirch's work this bit of history had been lost to the current era. This pattern of sleep is no longer the norm in developed countries, where artificial light extends the day, but anthropologists have observed a similar pattern of segmented sleep in some contemporary African tribes. Ekirch notes that the Tiv people of central Nigeria even use the same terms—first sleep and second sleep—used by the Europeans of times past.

Segmented Sleep May Be The Natural pattern: Several lines of evidence suggest that this archaic sleep pattern may, in fact, be the natural sleep pattern—the one most in tune with our inherent circadian rhythms and the natural environment. In the early 1990s, Thomas A. Wehr, MD, then a sleep researcher at the NIMH, and his colleagues reported that when 8 healthy men had their light/dark schedules shifted from their customary 16 hours of light, 8 hours of dark to one in which they were exposed to natural and artificial light for 10 hours each day and confined to a dark room for 14 hours each night (durations of light and dark similar to the natural durations of day and night in winter) a sleep pattern similar to that of the Pre-industrial Era developed. They slept in 2 bouts of about 4 hours each separated by 1 to 3 hours of quiet wakefulness. Subjects usually woke from their first bout of sleep during a period of rapid eye movement (REM) sleep, when dreaming is most likely. The second bout of sleep was usually lighter than the first, with less stage-4 (deep) and more REM sleep. Thus, when freed from the time constraints on night imposed by modern work schedules and artificial illumination, subjects reverted to the segmented sleep of earlier times.

Also suggesting that interrupted or segmented sleep comes to us naturally, many animals that are active during the day—including chimpanzees, chipmunks and giraffes—sleep at night in distinct bouts separated by several hours. In fact, Wehr points out, modern humans may be unique among animals in the extent to which their sleep is consolidated.

Dr. Wehr, now a Scientist Emeritus at the NIMH, thinks that our current sleep pattern, in which we fall asleep rapidly and expect to sleep (and often do) for an uninterrupted 7 or 8 hours, may be an artifact of both chronic sleep deprivation and artificial light. When the subjects of his experiment shifted from the "16-hour-days and 8-hour-night" (customary for them and for everyone else in developed countries who depend on artificial light) to the "natural winter" conditions of his experiment, they slept at first for 11 hours and then started sleeping for an average of 8.9 hours, compared to the 7.2 hours under ordinary conditions.

This together with other data suggests that our current schedules do not allow us the sleep that we require. Wehr also observed that when given 14 hours of darkness, it took subjects at bed rest about 2 hours to fall asleep, compared to the 15 minutes under usual conditions. He speculates that we may fall asleep so quickly because we are chronically sleep-deprived. Natural sleep, Wehr suggests, particularly during relatively long periods of darkness, is characterized by a long sleep latency and "interspersed with periods of wakefulness."

The discoveries of Ekirch and Wehr raise the possibility that segmented sleep is "normal" and as such they hold significant implications for both the understanding of sleep and the treatment of insomnia. But sleep specialists are, for the most part, unaware of these findings and have not yet incorporated them in clinical practice. Part of the reason lies with the fact that these discoveries have not been widely disseminated. Ekirch's book received a good number of deservedly positive reviews, but it is, after all history and is not at the top of most reading lists. While Wehr's sleep research is well known to sleep specialists, the thrust of his work has been on uncovering the mechanisms governing sleep. His discovery of segmented sleep was an unexpected, incidental finding from a study examining the influence of photoperiod on sleep and melatonin.

Also working against the clinical application of these findings is the extent to which they fly in the face of current thinking. The general public seems to regard 7 to 8 hours of unbroken sleep as our birthright; Anything less means that something is awry. Sleep specialists share this assumption. Sleep researcher J. Todd Arnedt, PhD, clinical assistant professor of psychiatry and neurology at the University of Michigan, acknowledges that the conventional approach to patients who cannot maintain sleep, and the one he uses, is to attempt to consolidate their sleep. He didn't know about the 2 bouts of sleep discovered by Ekirch and Wehr but, in light of that phenomenon, thinks that the conventional approach might not be the best one. He points out that how patients perceive their sleep determines to some extent how in fact they do sleep. He tries to get his patients with insomnia to stop seeing their sleep as problematic. When they can do that, whatever sleep loss they encounter becomes more tolerable. If patients perceived interrupted sleep as normal, he points out, they might experience less stress when they awaken at night and thus would fall back to sleep more easily.

Ekirch believes that the period of quiet wakefulness also offered a unique opportunity to contemplate dreams. People often awoke from a dreaming state and so were particularly likely to remember their dreams, and thus to gain access to an otherwise unavailable part of mental life. He believes that we may have lost something in our move to consolidated sleep.

Mary Carskadon, PhD, a sleep researcher at Brown University in Rhode Island, did not know of Ekirch's historical findings but did know of the segmented sleep pattern discovered by Wehr and of the fact that some animals take **"2 sleeps."** Considering these observations, she speculates that "maybe the brain can't keep you asleep for prolonged periods, and she wonders whether the archaic sleep pattern had some functional purpose." Like Ekirch, Carskadon believes that the change in sleep pattern "highlights something humanity might have lost in the hurly-burly times we live in today."

Much as we might envy the more relaxed sleep pattern of our forebears, we are unlikely to revert to it. As Carskadon points out, "It is hard to adapt to 2 bouts of sleep when you have to be at work at 8 am". She does feel, though, that it would benefit patients with interrupted sleep to tell them that such a sleep pattern may be natural.

The accountant troubled by broken sleep could well benefit from learning that the sleep pattern he finds so distressing may be more natural than the solid sleep he desires. And he should be told that in his nocturnal wakefulness he's far from alone. He is in the company not only giraffes and chipmunks but also of his ancestors and many of his contemporaries. If the usual measures don't suffice to give him the solid sleep he wants, tell him to savor the period before he returns to sleep. It is the time to meditate, have sex, and think about dreams. Or, as Wehr says, he can "just lie there and go back to sleep".

Review Posted by Dr. Paul Spector, MD [13]
Why You Can't Sleep Through the Night?

Dr. Thomas Wehr's Experiment: In the early 1990s Dr. Thomas Wehr, a sleep researcher at National Institute of Mental Health (NIMH) inadvertently stumbled on something that changed everything about sleep-wake cycle of humans.

Dr. Wehr selected healthy untroubled sleepers who were accustomed to 16 to 17 hours of daytime and 8 to 7 hours of nighttime for sleep, a routine that many of us live by or envy because we get less sleep. He exposed them to 10 hours of bright light per day (creating the daytime) and 14 hours of dark per day (creating the nighttime) and watched, and monitored everything that happened during their sleep. This ratio of light to dark (10:14) mimics the natural weather of a typical winter day in a temperate climate region. Initially, they slept for 11 hours per night, suggesting a chronic sleep deficit or sleep debt, and then settled into an average of 8.9 hours each night. By the fourth week Wehr saw something that wasn't supposed to happen in humans. They all developed a sleep pattern characterized by two sleep sessions (first sleep for 4 hours & second sleep for another 4 hours). Subjects tended to lie awake for 1 to 2 hours and then fall quickly asleep. After about 4 hours of solid sleep, they would awaken and spend 1 to 2 hours in a state of quiet wakefulness before a second 4-hour sleep period.

Researchers have replicated and expanded on Wehr's work. Several studies have taken subjects to deep underground bunkers free of any artificial light in order to observe our internal clock's rhythm. Again, they observe this biphasic pattern. Subjects sleep in two four-hour solid blocks separated by a couple hours of meditative quiet during which there is a remarkable surge of prolactin, unseen in modern humans. The participants report feeling so awake during the day that it is as if they experience true wakefulness for the first time.

In fact, a study of contemporary cultures across the globe reveals a wide spectrum of sleep habits. Some anthropologists now speak of three sleep cultures: monophasic cultures (the West, where one consolidated sleep period dominates), siesta cultures (where one afternoon nap is added in the afternoon, the word siesta meaning the sixth hour) and polyphasic cultures (China, Japan, India where multiple naps throughout the day of varying lengths are the norm).

Review Posted by Ethan Green [14]
What to Do When You Wake Up in The Night?
(When You Are Attacked By Middle-Of-The-Night Insomnia)

How often do you find yourself waking at a ridiculous hour, your mind flooded with every thought you'd rather not be having at that exact moment?

Whatever the reason is that you woke up, this barrage of unwanted thoughts then keeps you awake even longer. It is a vicious circle and one which I have personally been spun around in many times. You may experience this only occasionally or you may have a long-term inability to sleep throughout the night.

Sometimes called 'sleep maintenance insomnia' or 'middle-of-the-night insomnia', the good news is that it might not actually be as bad for you as you fear.

Why Does It Happen?
In this article I will be looking at some of the common reasons you may be waking up. Many of these reasons are things which you can then try to tackle. As with most forms of insomnia, it is often best seen as a symptom of another problem. And so the best approach is to work out what that first problem is and deal with it. In addition, I will look at a fascinating theory that suggests there is nothing wrong with sleeping in two phases.

The standard advice for adults has long been that 7-9 hours of solid sleep at night is best for the body and mind. But there is growing evidence that this may not necessarily be true. It may well be totally normal and even good for you to wake up in the night. If nothing else, it could be comforting to know that it is natural and not doing you any great harm. First let's have a look at some common reasons why you might be waking up.

Well, that is of course up to you to decide. But it may be a good idea to do something which is relaxing and not too stimulating for the brain.

♦ Doing relaxation exercises, reflecting and meditating may be a good way to spend the time for example.
♦ Alternatively, if you find that an hour or two is just too much time to lie awake in bed, then perhaps you could try experimenting with getting up and doing something quiet like reading or writing.
♦ The main thing is not to worry about it so long as it is not impacting on your quality of life and your well-being. Try not to allow this period of being awake to stress you out.
♦ Often the fear of not being able to fall asleep, of having insomnia or not functioning well the next day makes it harder to sleep.

Segmented Sleep by Dr. Roger Ekirch [15]

I came to discover that pre-industrial sleep was segmented. Unlike the seamless slumber we strive to achieve, sleep once commonly consisted of two major intervals, a "first sleep" and a "second sleep," bridged after midnight by an hour or more of wakefulness in which people did practically everything imaginable. They rose to perform chores, to tend to sick children, raid a neighbor's apple orchard. Others, remaining abed, recited prayers and pondered dreams. The 16th century French physician Laurent Joubert attributed the fecundity of manual laborers to early-morning intercourse "after the first sleep" when they "have more enjoyment" and "do it better." To judge from textual references as early as Homer's Odyssey, the prevailing mode of slumber for ages was biphasic. Virgil's Aeneid, composed in the first century BC, speaks of the "hour which terminates the first sleep, when the car of Night had as yet performed but half its course".

I also received emails from patients suffering from "middle-of-the-night" insomnia. Most expressed relief when they learned that their wakefulness was not necessarily abnormal — indeed, viewed from the cosmic perch of history, their slumber appeared quite natural. A growing number of doctors who treat insomniacs believe that knowledge of segmented sleep can help patients fall back asleep by easing their anxiety.

Sleep We Lost by Dr. Roger Ekirch [16]

"Our classic eight-hour-night only dates back to the invention of the light bulb in the late 1800s. Historians believe that before the dawn of electric lighting most people got plenty of sleep, and practiced what they call 'segmented sleep', snoozing for several hours in the first part of the night, when darkness fell, then waking in the middle of the night for a few hours of eating, drinking, praying, chatting with friends or maybe even canoodling, before ducking back under the covers again until morning. The arrival of electricity, argues sleep historian Dr. Roger Ekirch, led to later bedtimes and fewer hours of sleep overall."

"Dating well into the 18th century, two periods of wakefulness alternating with two shifts of sleep per 24 hours is normal. During this time period, it is common for people to pray, think, reflect on dreams, brew ale, and even visit neighbors in the middle of the night."

"The anthropologist and historian Dr. Roger Ekirch believes the largest contributing factor to the adoption of monophasic sleep (sleeping once a day) has been the widespread availability of artificial light since industrialization in the mid 19ᵗʰ century. He also says the arrival of electricity has triggered later bedtimes and fewer overall hours of rest. For centuries, polyphasic patterns dictated the 24-hour cycle. In the Middle Ages, adults typically slept in multiple segmented two to three hour periods, waking for stints of conscious restfulness, prayer, or sex before retiring again to slumber."

"<u>Computers, iPhones, Light Bulbs: they all attack our eyes with artificial light, tricking our body's biological clocks into living a perpetual high noon</u>.

Temporal disorientation is an unintended consequence of technological innovation. As a result we're missing out on true wakefulness and, in the process, creativity that sprouts from a brain that is properly rested. Waking up in the middle of the night? That's totally natural and it might do us some good, according to sleep historian Dr. Roger Ekirch of Virginia Tech. "Typically people went to bed at nine or 10 o'clock. They slept for three, at most, four hours, and then they rose" sometime after midnight to do "anything and everything imaginable," he says. Then people went back to bed until dawn to rise naturally with the morning light. That was before the gaslight proliferated in factories and homes in the early 1800s. Now, few of us know true night."

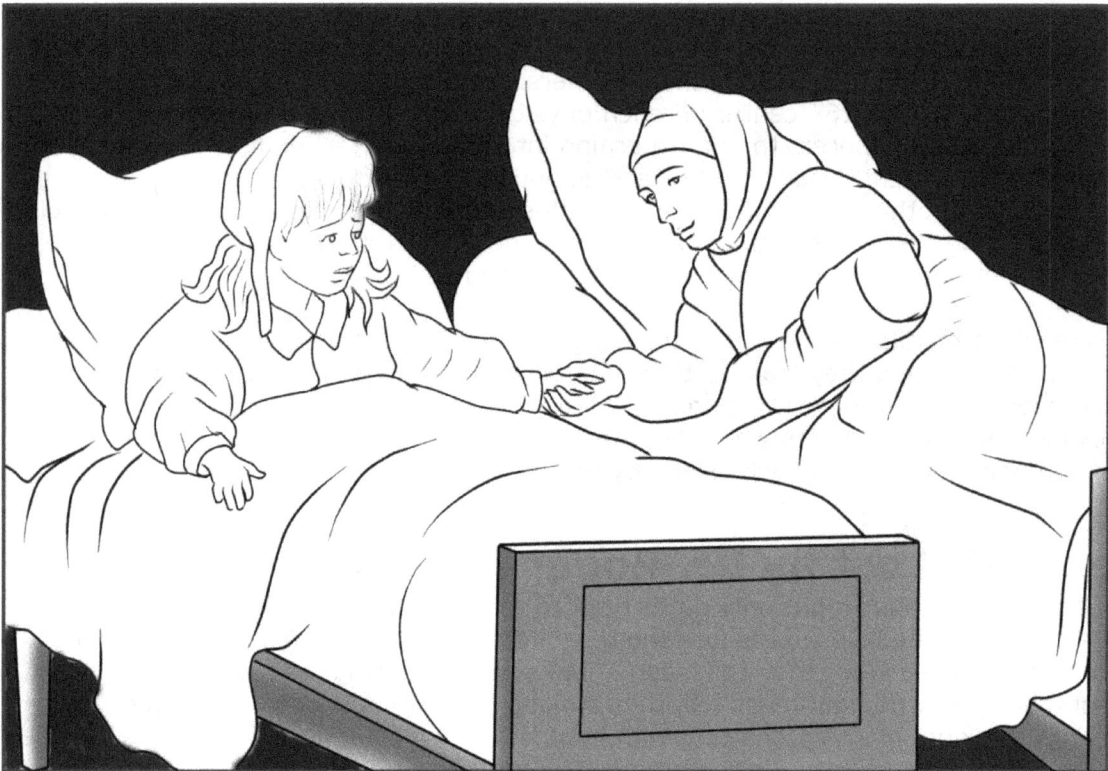

Figure 4.3 People became awake due to middle-of-the-night insomnia.

My "Questions and Answers" With Dr. Roger Ekirch on the Way We Sleep, and How It Has Changed Over the Centuries, Posted by Arianna Huffington [17]
June 24, 2015

Dr. Roger Ekirch is a professor of history at Virginia Tech and the author of 'At Day's Close: Night in Times Past'. He is also a leading scholar on segmented sleep -- the idea that for much of history people slept in two separate chunks separated by a waking period, as opposed to a single span of sleep. In answer to my questions, he shared his insights on "normal" insomnia, how technological advances have changed the way we sleep, and why in many ways we're living in a golden age of sleep.

1) How was the waking time between the two sleeps spent?
In myriad ways, from the spiritual to the profane, in addition to more mundane tasks such as rising to urinate, either in a chamber pot or, on mild evenings, outdoors. Fires needed to be tended or perhaps a tub of ale brewed. Virgil in the Aeneid wrote of women servants, after the first slumber, who ply the distaff by the winking light, and to their daily labor add the night. The sick were given potions and elixirs; whereas for the poor, the dead of night (midnight to three a.m.) was a prime time for poaching and petty theft so long as the moon, or "tattler," was not full. Orchards were pilfered and firewood filched. Still, most persons never left their beds, preferring instead to ponder dreams from which they were awakened. No other period afforded such a secluded interval of darkness to absorb fresh visions of solace, spirituality and self-revelation. There were also prayers to be recited when you awaken in the night. And no time was thought better for sexual intimacy if a couple wished to conceive children. A 16th century French physician ascribed the fecundity of rural peasants to early morning sexual intercourse "after the first sleep" when, he claimed, they "have more enjoyment" and "do it better."

2) How did the Industrial Revolution change how humans sleep?
The Revolution accentuated forces rooted in both technology and culture that transformed segmented sleep. As with other forms of biological change, the transition was lengthy and erratic. Nighttime slumber that had been "segmented," with a provenance as old as humankind, gradually, by the late 19th century, became compressed and consolidated throughout much of North America and Europe. Owing to a heightened sensitivity toward time, coupled with the growing importance of efficiency and productivity in daily life, sleep resembled, for many, a necessary evil best confined to a single interval -- "stealing a march, so to speak, on the day and on one's fellow human beings who are enjoying that second sleep," as a London writer advised. Proponents of "early rising," a very popular reform movement, urged parents to encourage children at an early age to arise after "their first sleep".

But even more decisive was the growing prevalence of artificial illumination within homes and businesses as well as on public streets -- first gas, followed in the late 1800s by electric lighting. As scientific research has shown, modern lighting can have a profound physiological effect upon sleep. Just a few hours of exposure can reset the circadian pacemaker controlling the flow of hormones and changes in body functions that have daily rhythms. Then, too, the dissemination of artificial lighting led to later bedtimes and sleep that was deeper, more compressed, and capable of being taken in a single interval. By the early 20th century, if not earlier, most people exhibited an unquestioning adherence to seamless slumber.

3) Do you believe we have evolved past a pattern of segmented sleep, or are our bodies struggling against us when we try to sleep in one chunk of time? How do modern sleep disorders relate to all this?

If anything, the changes in technology and cultural attitudes responsible for the decline of segmented sleep have grown more powerful in the wake of the 19th century. Short of retreating to an ill-lit cabin in Yukon, there is no turning back. That said, a significant segment of the population in the United States and abroad yet experience a biphasic pattern of sleep. Over ten per cent of Americans reportedly suffer from "middle-of-the-night" (MOTN) insomnia, the most common variety of sleeplessness whereby they have difficulty in falling asleep and lie awake in the night for an hour or more. To both, their frustration and that of their physicians', there appears to be no explicable reason for their wakefulness. Many patients, I have been told, regard themselves as abnormal, which only heightens their anxiety, thereby accentuating their inability to sleep. But there is strong historical evidence that many insomniacs may, in fact, be experiencing this older, more natural pattern of segmented slumber.

Notably, middle-of-the-night insomnia was not a problem before the late 1800s. Medical texts as early as the 16th century regarded the interval of wakefulness separating first from second sleep as utterly normal and, hence, unworthy of discussion except for affording a preferred time for ingesting medicine, engaging in sex, and shifting from one side of the body to another to aid digestion. Fitful sleep, whether caused by sickness, bugs, or inclement weather, was not confused with wakefulness between the first and second sleep. In fact, not until the turn of the 19th century and sleep's consolidation did physicians view nocturnal awakening as an illness requiring medication.

What about individuals today who awaken in the middle of the night while the rest of us sleep seamlessly? Some who are prone to nocturnal awakenings may possess circadian rhythms capable of withstanding the impact of artificial lighting, or are otherwise disposed to resist the transition to consolidation. Further, as David Neubauer at Johns Hopkins has speculated, consolidated sleep, as an artificial invention of modern life, may be inherently unstable and, thus, all the more vulnerable to disruption. It also stands to reason that the transition from segmented sleep, dominant in all likelihood since time immemorial, would take longer than just one or even two centuries to run its course.

4) Based on your knowledge of the history of sleep, what steps can people take today to improve their sleep?

Two things. First, despite rising complaints of insomnia, we should delight in the fact that for most of us, the opportunity to enjoy deep, restful sleep has never been better, thanks to improvements in home construction, heating, and medical care, not least aspirin and other modern analgesics. Notwithstanding nostalgic stereotypes of repose in simpler times, slumber before the Industrial Revolution was frequently disturbed, a consequence in that pre-penicillin age of rampant illness as well as depression and mental anxiety arising from hardships and fears, both real and imaginary. A diary kept by the Connecticut colonist Hannah Heaton recounts numerous nocturnal battles with Satan, resulting in frequent loss of rest. Primitive living conditions magnified such woes, from frigid temperatures, noise, and leaky roofs to bed bugs, lice, and fleas, the unholy trinity of pre-industrial entomology.

Why, then, is there a modern epidemic of sleep deprivation? Certainly one explanation for this paradox lies in the mistaken belief that sleep can be shortchanged without having to pay for the consequences.

By burning the candle at both ends -- rising early for work after retiring around midnight, if not later -- we have come to expect six or seven hours of undisturbed rest. Ironically, the less time allowed for sleep, the more we have come to demand of it, hoping that expensive bedding and sleeping pills will compensate for our high wattage lifestyle. And then to cope with our exhaustion during the day, we look, often in vain, to such popular expedients as power naps and caffeinated beverages -- not just coffee but high energy drinks. In truth, unlike our ancestors, many of us have only ourselves to blame, all the more if we remain on our computers late at night, which like other sources of sensory stimulation such as video games and television, are detrimental to fostering sleep.

Second, people who suffer from middle-of-the-night insomnia should understand, from an historical perspective, that their sleep may well be utterly normal. Their circadian rhythms may vibrate to an older, more natural tuning fork. That is slight consolation perhaps, but at the very least this knowledge should alleviate their anxiety at night, not to mention the psychological consequences of thinking oneself abnormal or, worse, a "freak."

My Questions and Answers With Insomnia Expert
Dr. Gregg Jacobs, Posted by Arianna Huffington [17]
March 31, 2015

Dr. Gregg Jacobs is an insomnia specialist at the Sleep Disorders Center at the UMass Memorial Medical Center and the author of 'Say Good Night to Insomnia'. He is also an American film director, assistant director, producer and screenwriter. In answer to several questions, he shared his insights on how human sleep patterns have changed over time, what are healthier and more effective alternatives to sleeping pills, and how to reverse our worst sleep habits and behaviors.

Describe your research on insomnia?

I have a longstanding interest in the relationship between the mind and health. My doctoral research, which assessed the ability of the mind to control physiology, showed that it was possible to use deep relaxation techniques to voluntarily produce brain wave patterns that were identical to the initial stages of sleep. My postdoctoral research at Harvard Medical School included research on the meditative practices of Tibetan monks. This research, conducted in a Tibetan monastery in Sikkim under the auspices of the Dalai Lama, revealed that advanced Tibetan monks possess remarkable control over their brain waves and physiology. This led to my efforts to develop a safe, drug-free intervention for insomnia, called cognitive behavioral therapy for insomnia (CBT-I), over the past 30 years at the Harvard and University of Massachusetts medical schools. This research culminated in a landmark study, funded by the National Institutes of Health, showing that CBT-I is more effective than Ambien. Because few people have access to CBT-I, my more recent efforts have focused on making CBT-I widely available in an inexpensive, practical format through my website, cbtforinsomnia.com. Numerous studies have recently demonstrated that internet-based CBT-I can be delivered as effectively as face-to-face CBT-I and is more practical and cost-effective.

You've discussed the history of segmented sleep. Do you believe we have evolved past this pattern, or are our bodies struggling against us when we try to sleep in one chunk of time? How does insomnia relate to this?

Research suggests that we may have displayed a polyphasic (i.e., multiple periods) sleep pattern for virtually all of our evolution until the recent advent of nighttime lighting. Prior to that, humans likely went to sleep soon after dusk and awakened at dawn in longer sleep periods that consisted of alternating bouts of sleep and wakefulness. This non-continuous sleep pattern is characteristic of virtually all mammals and is also the pattern we experience early and late in life. It is only in adult life, and the last 350 years of human history, that a more consolidated nocturnal sleep pattern is apparent. However, many adults still experience polyphasic sleep in the form of insomnia, and regular intervals of waking are still experienced in normal sleepers today, as evidenced by 6 to 12 brief awakenings per night (which most of us don't recall, for they are too short). Evidently, this polyphasic sleep pattern lies dormant in our physiology, met an evolutionary need, and therefore may be adaptive rather than a sleep disorder.

In segmented sleep, how was the waking time between the two sleeps spent?

In prehistoric times, it may have been spent tending to the fire, being vigilant for predators, in deep relaxation, for creativity and problem solving, and a channel of communication between dreams and waking life. Historical accounts suggest it was used for sexual activity and socializing, reading and writing, praying, meditating on dreams, or tending to the fire in the cold months.

Tell me about cognitive behavioral therapy, or CBT. How does this treatment for insomnia compare with other methods like sleeping pills? What successes have you seen among your patients, and how can others incorporate the strategies into their sleep habits?

CBT-I is the most effective psychology-based treatment for a health problem and has consistently been proven to be the most effective first-line treatment for chronic insomnia. It improves sleep in 75 to 80 percent of insomnia patients and reduces or eliminates sleeping pill use in 90 percent of patients. It is so effective that I am surprised if my patients do not report improvement in sleep, or a reduction or elimination of sleeping pills, from CBT-I. And in three studies published in major medical journals that directly compared CBT with sleeping pills, including my study at Harvard Medical School, CBT-I was more effective than sleeping pills. CBT-I also has no side effects and maintains improvements in sleep long-term, and new research shows that CBT-I doubles the improvement rates of depression compared with antidepressant medication alone in depressed patients with insomnia.

In contrast to CBT-I, sleeping pills do not greatly improve sleep. Objectively, newer-generation sleeping pills such as Ambien are no more effective than a placebo. Subjectively, they only increase total sleep time, and reduce the time it takes to fall asleep, by about 10 minutes. Furthermore, these small to moderate short-term improvements in sleep are often outweighed by significant side effects and risks, particularly in older adults. These include impairment of alertness, driving, and learning and memory (including sleep-dependent memory consolidation); increased mortality risk, as shown in almost two dozen scientific studies; and dependence, addiction, and activation of the same neurobiological pathways involved in drugs of abuse.

CBT-I is based on the idea that some individuals react to short-term insomnia (usually caused by stress) by worrying about sleep loss. After a few weeks of lying awake at night, frustrated and anxious about insomnia, they start to anticipate not sleeping and become apprehensive about going to bed. They soon learn to associate the bed with sleeplessness and frustration; consequently, the bed quickly becomes a learned cue for wakefulness and insomnia. As a result, they begin to engage in these types of maladaptive sleep habits, thoughts and behaviors that exacerbate insomnia that must be changed with CBT-I (sleeping pills are marginally effective because they do not change these behaviors):

- Negative, distorted thoughts and beliefs about insomnia such as "I must get eight hours of sleep" or "I did not sleep a wink last night"
- Going to bed too early or sleeping too late and spending excessive time in bed
- Irregular rising times
- Trying to control sleep rather than letting it happen
- Lying awake in bed, frustrated and tense
- Using the bed and bedroom for activities other than sleep
- Use of electronic devices before bedtime

Don't Be Bothered Too Much By Interrupted Sleep! Just Get Used To It, And Cope With It!

The number of hours each adult sleeps varies from person to person. On average most adults need around 8 hours of good night's sleep. As a person grows older, the sleep pattern changes and if the person monitors and understands carefully the sleep pattern and by reading and researching, he/she could easily treat the sleep difficulties at home without seeing a specialist and without ever taking any prescription sleeping pills.

Insomnia is the state of being awake when a person wants to sleep and maintain the sleep for longer periods of time to the full satisfaction. Depending on the severity, there are several types of insomnia such as acute insomnia (short-term insomnia), chronic insomnia (long-term insomnia), learned insomnia, primary insomnia, onset insomnia, middle insomnia, terminal insomnia and hypersomnia. For detailed descriptions of all types of insomnia, please see CHAPTER 3.

Many people panic if there are attacked by the middle-of-the-night insomnia or by interrupted sleep and make appointments with sleep specialists and go on taking prescription sleeping pills because of the lack of education. They are not aware of the fact that middle-of-the-night insomnia is a natural sleep pattern and can be treated by simply being accustomed to it. Several hundred years ago before the electricity was discovered, our ancestors used to sleep with one or more interruptions, and used to live up to their full satisfaction with refreshed mood. Historian Dr. Roger Ekirch [3], after conducting 16 years of research, reported that our ancestors used to sleep in two segments. During interruption between the two segments, people were accustomed to go to bathrooms, visit neighbors, participate in conversation, read books and pray collectively, and some couples would make sex during the interval. After the interval, they were accustomed to enjoy the second segment of sleep, and would wake up in the morning completely refreshed.

RECOMMENDATION ON MIDDLE-OF-THE-NIGHT INSOMNIA (by Dr. RK)

If you are suffering from middle-of-the-night insomnia, refer to the main article of this course and read the Instruction # 24 "How to treat Middle-of-the-Night Insomnia," and follow the treatment method explained there (there are 9 tips provided by Dr. RK). Please do not practice "Segmented Sleep" intentionally. If you are attacked by middle-of-the-night insomnia, don't worry, but just treat it peacefully in a relaxed mood as if everything was normal. Living alone in the **DARK ROOM (PITCH-BLACK ROOM)** during the nighttime, without any kind of light (a battery-powered lamp can be used during walking only), would significantly help improve your sleep and combat chronic insomnia. Do not take sleeping pills. They are unnecessary and they don't work. Your brain is capable to secrete as much melatonin as your body needs and to make you sleep. The spontaneous melatonin production by the pineal gland located in your brain is the key to attaining a good night's sleep.

REFERENCES

1. THOMAS WEHR'S RESEARCH STUDY PUBLISHED IN WIKIPEDIA.Org
Middle-of-the-Night Insomnia Could Be A Normal Sleep Pattern.
https://en.wikipedia.org/wiki/Thomas_Wehr

2. In Short Photoperiods, Human Sleep is Biphasic
Author: THOMAS A. WEHR, Journal of Sleep Research
Volume 1, Issue 2, pages 103–107, June 1992
Article first published online: 20 JAN 2009
DOI: 10.1111/j.1365-2869.1992.tb00019.x
© 1992 European Sleep Research Society.
a. https://www.ncbi.nlm.nih.gov/pubmed/10607034

b. http://onlinelibrary.wiley.com/doi/10.1111/j.1365-2869.1992.tb00019.x/abstract

c. http://onlinelibrary.wiley.com/doi/10.1111/j.1365-2869.1992.tb00019.x/abstract;jsessionid=024630F96609E3CDE5BD545430BCBE87.d03t03

3. DR. ROGER EKIRCH's Book, At Day's Close: Night in Times Past, Paperback, 480 pages, Published by W. W. Norton & Company, October 17, 2006.

4. Segmented Sleep (from Wikipedia)
https://en.wikipedia.org/wiki/Segmented_sleep (old link, broken)
https://en.wikipedia.org/wiki/Biphasic_and_polyphasic_sleep

5. Review Posted by Susannah Ottaway: DR. ROGER EKIRCH, At Day's Close: Night in Times Past, 2005, 447 pages.
https://muse.jhu.edu/article/212756

6. Review Posted by Ian Pindar, DR. ROGER EKIRCH, At Day's Close: Night in Times Past.
https://www.theguardian.com/books/2005/jul/30/featuresreviews.guardianreview8

7. Dr. CraigM. Koslofsky Ph.D.,Department of History, University of Illinois at Chicago, Illinois, USA.
http://www.history.illinois.edu/people/koslof

8. Dr. Craig Koflofsky's Book: Evening's Empire: A History of the Night in Early Modern Europe, Amazon.com, Cambridge and New York: Cambridge University Press, 2011.
http://www.amazon.com/Evenings-Empire-History-Studies-European/dp/0521721067

9. Review Posted by Prof. Joad Raymond (Professor of English Literature at the University of East Anglia), About the Book Dr. Craig Koflofsky, Evening's Empire: A History of the Night in Early Modern Europe, Published in History Today Volume 62 Issue 2 February 2012.
http://www.historytoday.com/blog/2012/02/history-night-early-modern-europe

10. Review Posted by Adam McDowell, Rest assured: There's Nothing Wrong with Segmented Sleep, Special to National Post | July 16, 2012 6:20 PM ET.
http://news.nationalpost.com/life/rest-assured-theres-nothing-wrong-with-segmented-sleep

11. Review Posted by Stephanie Hegarty, The Myth of an Eight-Hour Sleep, BBC World Service, February 22, 2012.
http://www.bbc.com/news/magazine-16964783

12. Review Posted by Dr. Walter A. Brown, MD, Broken Sleep May Be Natural Sleep, March 1, 2007.
http://www.depressionforums.org/sleep/2512-broken-sleep-may-be-natural-sleep

13. Review Posted by Dr. Paul Spector, MD
Why You Can't Sleep Through the Night, Nov 21, 2012.
http://www.huffingtonpost.com/paul-spector-md/why-you-might-have-troubl_b_1883811.html

14. Review Posted by Ethan Green, Waking Up In the Middle-of-the-night May Be Normal, August 1, 2016.
http://www.nosleeplessnights.com/do-we-really-need-to-sleep-all-through-the-night/

15. Segmented Sleep by Dr. Roger Ekirch, Harper's Magazine, August 2013.
http://harpers.org/archive/2013/08/segmented-sleep/

16. Sleep We Lost by Prof. Dr. Roger Ekirch, Department of History, VirginiaTech, USA.
http://www.history.vt.edu/Ekirch/sleepcommentary.html

17. My "Questions and Answers" With Dr. Roger Ekirch on the Way We Sleep, and How It's Changed Over the Centuries, Posted by Arianna Huffington, June 24, 2015.
https://www.huffingtonpost.com/arianna-huffington/my-q-and-a-with-roger-ekirch_b_7649554.html

18. My "Questions and Answers" With Insomnia Expert Dr. Gregg Jacobs, Posted by Arianna Huffington, March 31, 2015.
http://www.huffingtonpost.com/arianna-huffington/gregg-jacobs-insomnia_b_6978110.html

19. Gregg D. Jacobs (Author), Herbert Benson (Introduction),
Say Good Night to Insomnia: The Six-Week, Drug-Free Program Developed At Harvard Medical School Paperback – Sep 15 2009.
https://www.amazon.ca/Say-Good-Night-Insomnia-Drug-Free/dp/0805089586/ref=sr_1_1?ie=UTF8&qid=1493227790&sr=8-1&keywords=gregg+jacobs

CHAPTER 5: CIRCADIAN RHYTHMS & BIOLOGICAL CLOCK

TABLE OF CONTENTS

CIRCADIAN RHYTHMS

The word circadian is taken from the Latin language in which circa means approximately, and diem means the day. Therefore the meaning of the word circadian is "the approximate daily cycle".

Your sleep-wake cycle is dictated by the circadian rhythm. The circadian rhythms of humans are the biological cycles of many different processes that happen simultaneously over a time span of about 24 hours as shown in the diagram below. [1, 2]

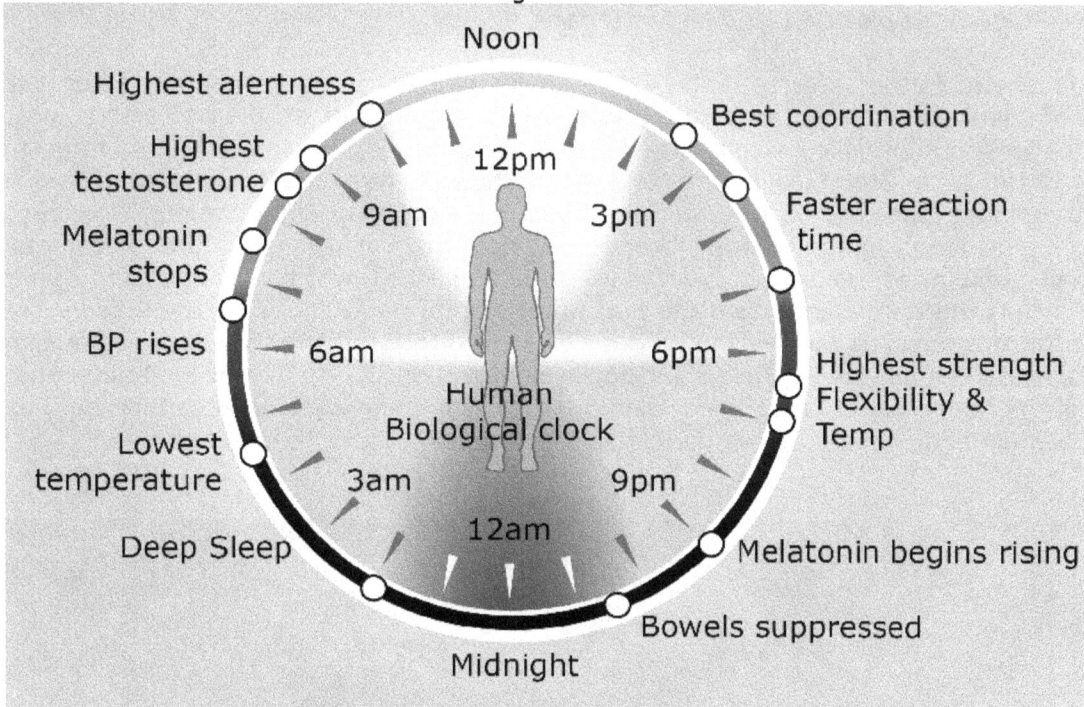

Figure 5.1 Most common Ccrcadian rhythms in a 24-hour cycle.

Here Are Some Most Common Circadian Rhythms During a 24-Hour Cycle:

- 6 am — AM Cortisol & BP increase in the morning to wake your brain and body.
- 6:45 am — Sharpest rise in blood pressure takes place.
- 7:30 am — MELATONIN PRODUCTION STOPS SO THAT YOU BECOME AWAKE.
- 8:30 am — Bowel movement likely to start, and you feel like discharging a stool.
- 9 am — Sex hormone "testosterone" production peaks.
- 10 am — Mental alertness peaks (highest) so you can focus on working hard.
- 12 pm — It is lunch time, so you feel hungry.
- 2:30 pm — Best coordination to be productive in your work.
- 3:30 pm — Fastest reaction time.
- 5 pm — Greatest cardiovascular efficiency and muscle strength.
- 6 pm — It is dinner time, so you feel hungry again.
- 6:30 pm — Highest blood pressure, strength & flexibility.
- 7:00 pm — Highest body temperature.
- 9 pm — MELATININ PRODUCTION STARTS SO THAT YOU BECOME SLEEPY.
- 2:30 am — Bowel movement suppresses.
- 12 am — Midnight, everybody is sleeping including you.
- 2 am — You fall into deep sleep. MELATONIN LEVEL PEAKS.
- 2:30 am — Lowest body temperature.

The aforementioned times not being exact merely display the general patterns of the circadian rhythms. The exact times of your circadian rhythms vary based on daylight, your habits, and other factors related to the nature where you live and your body's biological response to its environment.

OUR PLANET EARTH, BY MAKING ONE ROTATION EVERY 24 HOURS, AND BY REVOLVING AROUND THE SUN, CREATES DAYTIME AND NIGHTTIME.

We are living in a universe that includes planets, stars, galaxies, the intergalactic space, the smallest subatomic particles, and all matter and energy.

Earth is located in the universe in the Virgo Supercluster of galaxies. A supercluster is a group of galaxies held together by gravity. Within this supercluster, planet Earth is located in a smaller group of galaxies called the Local Group, and Earth is in the second largest galaxy of the Local Group, called the Milky Way. The Milky Way is a large spiral galaxy. Here the planet Earth is a part of the Solar System - a group of eight planets, "Mercury, Venus, Earth, Mars, Jupiter, Saturn, Uranus and Neptune," as well as numerous comets and many smaller asteroids and dwarf planets such as Pluto, which orbit the Sun. Sun is a star. Earth is the third planet from the Sun (after Mercury and Venus) in the Solar System. The Earth rotates on its own axis in an anticlockwise direction. And the Earth at the same time revolves around the Sun in an anticlockwise direction. All the major 8 planets, and most of the minor planets (asteroids) also orbit the Sun in an anticlockwise direction, except a few planets and comets orbit in the clockwise direction (opposite direction). [3, 4]

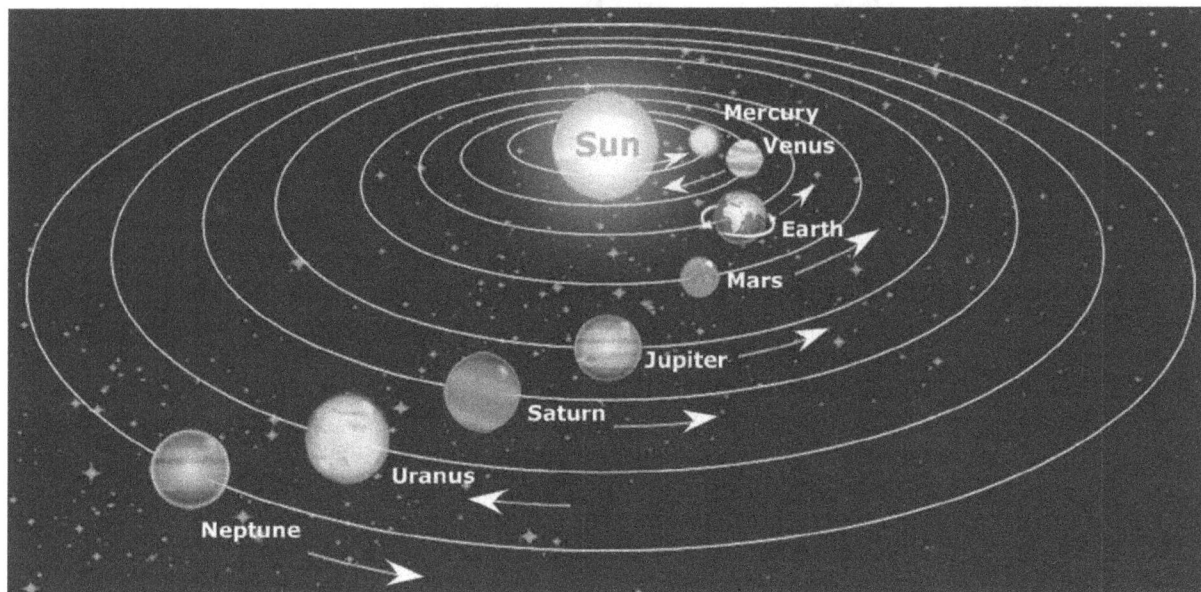

Figure 5.2 Our solar system (a group of 8 planets).

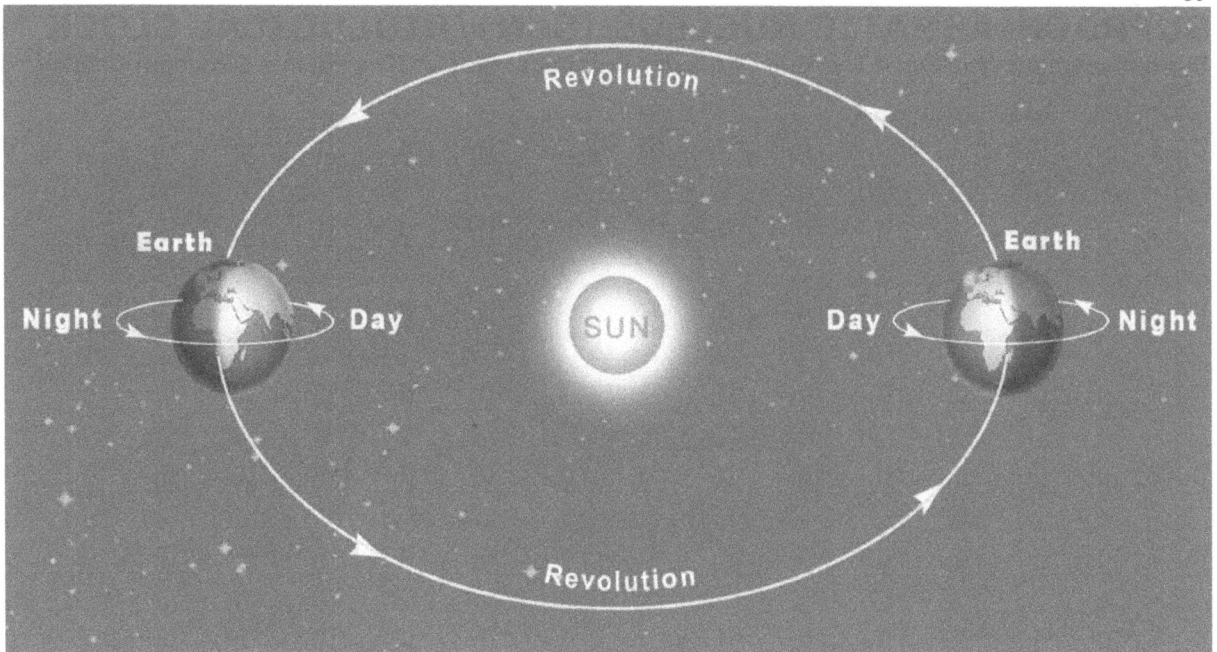

Figure 5.3   The Earth, by rotating on its own axis and by revolving around the Sun, creates day & night.

The Earth rotates on its own axis from the west towards east by turning in the counter-clockwise direction, and at the same time revolves around the sun. It takes for the Earth about 24 hours to rotate on it own axis by forming the day and night (approximately twelve hours for the day and 12 hours for the night). When the earth rotates on its own axis, half of the earth faces the sun, light rays emit from the sun and we call it the daytime, and the other half of earth that does not face the sun would not receive the light rays from the sun and stays in the dark, and we call it the nighttime. The people living on one half of the earth facing the sun receive light from the sun and feel that it is daytime, and the people living on the other half of the earth, not facing the sun, live in the dark by not receiving the light from the sun, and feel it is nighttime. Thus the earth rotates about its own axis every day, forming the day and night, and at the same time it revolves around the sun. In general, the earth takes 365.25 days (1 year) to revolve around the sun while continuing to rotate about its own axis. [5, 6]

As the Earth rotates around its axis in 24 hours by creating day and night, the circadian rhythms take place in a roughly 24-hour cycle depending on the amount of light and the amount of darkness the human body receives through the retinas of both their eyes. The rhythms could be physical, mental and behavioral. [7]

SUPRACHIASMATIC NUCLEUS (SCN)/BIOLOGICAL CLOCK
Suprachiasmatic Nucleus = The Brain's Master Biological Clock = The Brain's Circadian Clock

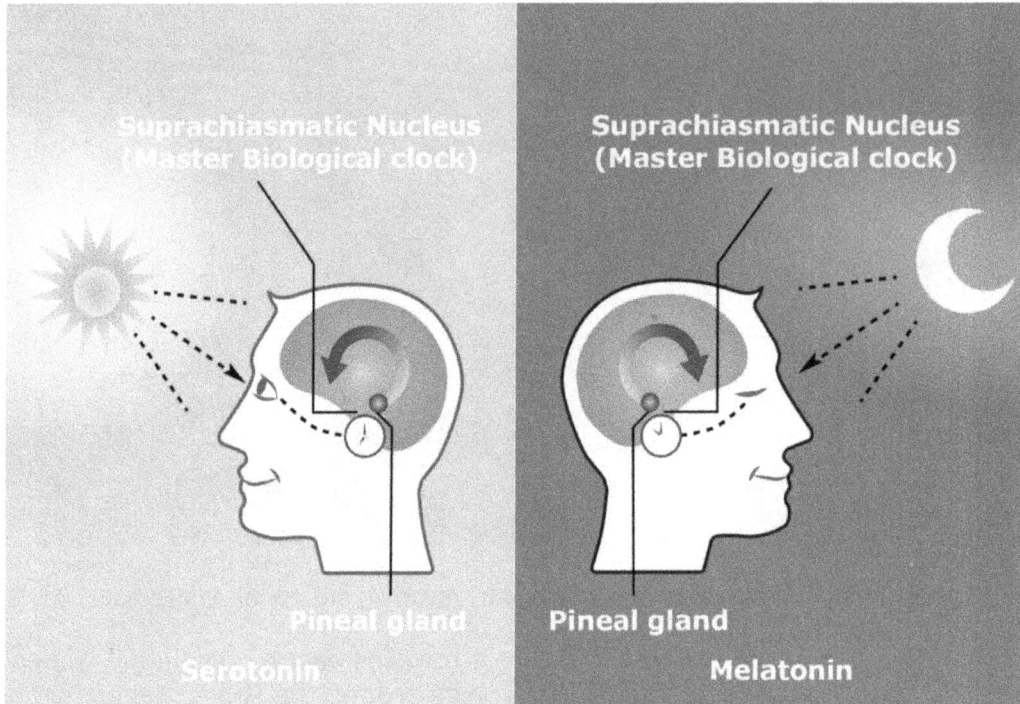

Figure 5.4 Sunshine promotes serotonin and moonlight promotes melatonin.

The trillions of cells in the human body are divided into many interacting groups, and into each group of molecules in the cells is embedded a biological clock to perform their functions in a rhythmic order synchronizing each other. These biological clocks drive our circadian rhythms. A circadian rhythm refers to a pattern of various biological functions that take place in an inherent cycle of 24 hours, by controlling and regulating the sleep-wake cycle, body temperature, blood pressure, digestion, metabolism, hormone release, hunger, fertility, mood and many other physiological conditions.

The hypothalamus is the portion of the brain that contains a number of small nuclei with a variety of functions. The suprachiasmatic nucleus (SCN), embedded in the hypothalamus of the brain (just above the optic chiasm) containing about 20,000 nerve cells, coordinates all the individual biological clocks so that they are all in sync, and acts as the brain's master biological clock or the brain's circadian clock.

It receives information from the retinas of both eyes, depending on the amount of light and amount of darkness in the environment, and acts accordingly to activate the pineal gland to produces melatonin. Melatonin is a sleep hormone released by the pineal gland into the bloodstream. [8, 9]

The suprachiasmatic nucleus (SCN) of the hypothalamus, by representing the master biological clock, regulates the circadian rhythms. All our body functions are directly tied to these individual biological clocks. If the individual biological clocks fail to function properly, we develop disorders and diseases such as insomnia, diabetes, depression and others. Even the effectiveness of prescription drugs and supplements greatly depends on how these biological clocks function. [9]

The individual biological clocks and the master biological clock are automatically adjusted daily by the amount of light or darkness received by the retinas of both eyes. In other words, the body's biological processes take place, depending on the position of the Earth against the sun.

This kind of activity automatically controls and regulates the circadian rhythms. Your master biological clock, believe it or not, is capable to wake you up in the morning every day at the same time without any alarm clock.

As the master biological clock is reset every day, by taking appropriate action as outlined in this course (by living in the dark during the night after 7 pm and by exposing yourself to sunlight and bright artificial lights during the day after 7 am), it is possible to reverse circadian rhythm disorder in a single day.

ALL YOU GOT TO DO IS: Reset your master biological clock if you suffer from insomnia. You can do it in one day or in one month. Right on the first night when you start treating the circadian rhythm disorder following carefully the instructions outlined in this course by turning off the lights in the evening and by living in the dark, you would notice yourself yawning excessively and you will feel like sleeping. Check it out with your own experience!

PINEAL GLAND AND ITS FUINCTIONS [10, 11, 12, 13, 14, 15, 16]

The **pineal gland** is a tiny pea-sized and cone-shaped endocrine gland situated deep inside the brain. In Latin, pinea means "pine cone." This tiny gland secretes the hormone melatonin. [10] The pineal gland produces the serotonin and also its derivative melatonin. The hormone melatonin influences the sexual development, sleep-wake cycles, and seasonal functions. That means melatonin secreted by the pinal gland helps regulate body's internal master biological clock and circadian rhythms such as sleep-wake cycles. In other words, it is melatonin that directs your internal clock, the one that allows you to wake up about the same time every morning without an alarm clock.

Serotonin and melatonin have opposite functions: Serotonin stimulates the mood during the day whereas the melatonin is responsible to inform a person that it is time to sleep.

Serotonin, the precursor to melatonin, is secreted when sunlight strikes the retinas, and is mostly responsible to create good mood, appetite and cognitive functions, feelings of well-being and happiness in the summer months. Lower amounts of serotonin in the winter months could cause depression. But during the summer months, your body could produce more than sufficient amount of serotonin and store it for future use in the winter months. So it is very important to take advantage of the summer months, exposing your body to the sun as much as you could. The brighter the sunlight and the longer a person is exposed to it, the greater the amount of serotonin produced by the pineal gland. The blue light and UV light from sunshine are essential for the production of serotonin. Sunlight has the UV light, which by absorbing through your skin produces Vitamin-D. Vitamin-D plays many roles in your body, including promoting serotonin production. In order to get enough serotonin, sun exposure is of utmost importance. Several scientific experiments in rats showed that the rate of production of serotonin by the brain is directly related to the prevailing duration of bright sunlight. [13]

When the daylight fades away and it gets dark outside, the retinas of both eyes detect the lower intensity of light, and send signals to the suprachiasmatic nucleus (SCN) of the hypothalamus, which in turn signals the pineal gland to start the melatonin production and to drop the body temperature so that a person would prepare to sleep. Then the pineal gland stops the secretion of serotonin, and starts secreting the hormone melatonin. The duration of melatonin secretion each day is directly proportional to the length of the night.

The average blood levels of melatonin throughout the day mirrors typical circadian rhythms. Low amounts of melatonin correspond to heightened alertness. High amounts of melatonin relate to periods of drowsiness and sleep. Blood levels of melatonin are essentially undetectable during daytime, but rise sharply during the dark. [13]

During the winter months in some countries with shorter daytime hours and longer nighttime hours, the secretion of serotonin and melatonin becomes unbalanced, and as a result the total amount of serotonin in a given day decreases dramatically, thereby affecting the mood and sleep patterns. When spring comes back, daytime hours increase and sunlight triggers the serotonin levels, and people experience great relief. [16]

FUNCTIONS OF SEROTONIN [12]
Serotonin influences the majority of brain cells either directly or indirectly. Listed below are some important functions of serotonin:

a. Bowel function: About 80% of serotonin is found in the gastrointestinal tract where it regulates bowel function and movements. It also controls appetite while consuming a meal.
b. Mood: Serotonin plays a major role in the brain cells by improving a person's mood, anxiety, and happiness. Some illicit mood-altering drugs such as Ecstasy and LSD cause a massive rise in serotonin levels.
c. Blood Clotting: Serotonin is immediately released by platelets whenever there is a wound. Serotonin plays a role in vasoconstriction (narrowing of the tiny arteries), and reduces the blood flow and aids the formation of blood clots.
d. Nausea: When you eat something that is toxic or irritating, more serotonin is produced in the gut to increase transit time and expel the irritant in diarrhea.
e. Bone density: Studies have shown that a persistent high level of serotonin in the bones can lead to an increase in osteoporosis.
f. Depression: Decreased levels of serotonin may cause depression.

PRODUCTION OF SEROTONIN AND MELATONIN [11, 14, 18]
Serotonin is also called neurotransmitter and is derived from the amino acid tryptophan. In the pineal gland, serotonin is acetylated and then methylated to yield melatonin when the retinas of the eyes sense darkness during the night.

Serotonin is produced in the gut (intestines) as well as in the brain by pineal gland. Between 80% and 90% of the serotonin can be found in the gastrointestinal tract. The remaining 10% to 20% is produced by pineal gland situated in the brain. Sunlight promotes serotonin production and darkness promotes melatonin production.

THE PRECURSORS FOR SEROTONIN AND MELATONIN: Our bodies (either the intestine or the pineal gland) do not produce serotonin or melatonin out of thin air. In order to produce serotonin and/or melatonin, the brain needs an amino acic called tryptophan that cannot be created by the body. We can only obtain tryptophan from our diet in protein-rich foods such as meat, fish, dairy products, egg whites, all animal products, nuts and seeds, legumes, and in some fruits as well.

The cell clusters in the Suprachiasmatic Nucleus (SCN) cause the pineal gland to manufacture and secrete both hormones, serotonin and melatonin, depending on the time of the 24-hour biological clock. Some specific brain chemicals and neural pathways in the pineal gland are responsible for regulating the mood and human behavior. [11] The pineal gland by functioning appropriately based on the climate and time of the day or night, produces both serotonin and melatonin. The pineal gland does not secrete melatonin during the day. Daytime and sunshine inhibit the production of melatonin. The pineal gland begins producing melatonin in the evening.

The amino acid tryptophan from the blood is first converted into serotonin in the pineal gland (this reaction is light dependent), which is then converted into the hormone melatonin (N-acetyl-5-methoxytryptamine). When the amino acid tryptophan enters the brain cells, a specialized enzyme helps convert the tryptophan into 5-hydroxy tryptophan, which is further reacts with another enzyme to form a neurotransmitter called serotonin. Some of this serotonin by reacting with another enzyme called N-acetyl-transferase is converted into a substance called N-acetyl serotonin. The pineal gland then with the help of another enzyme converts N-acetyl serotonin into the final product melatonin. [11, 14, 18] The pineal gland then secretes melatonin whenever it is appropriate, mostly during the nighttime, in order to signal the body that it is time to sleep.

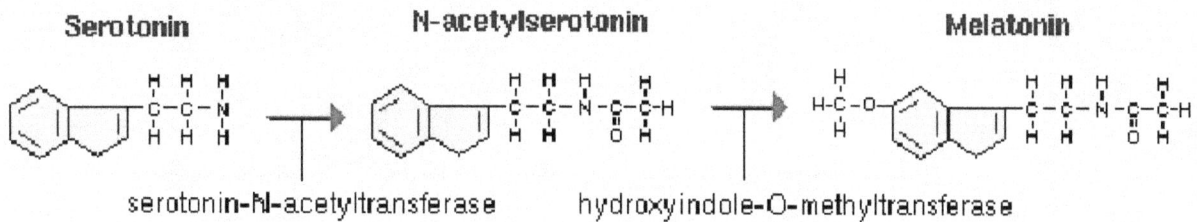

Figure 5.5 The chemical structure of serotonin and melatonin.

MELATONIN CHART [17, 18, 19, 20]

The rise and fall of melatonin level in the bloodstream during a typical day is depicted in a table and in a chart below. It is important to note that the melatonin levels rise sharply after 8 pm, and reach the peak between 2 am and 4 am, during which time a person goes into deep sleep.

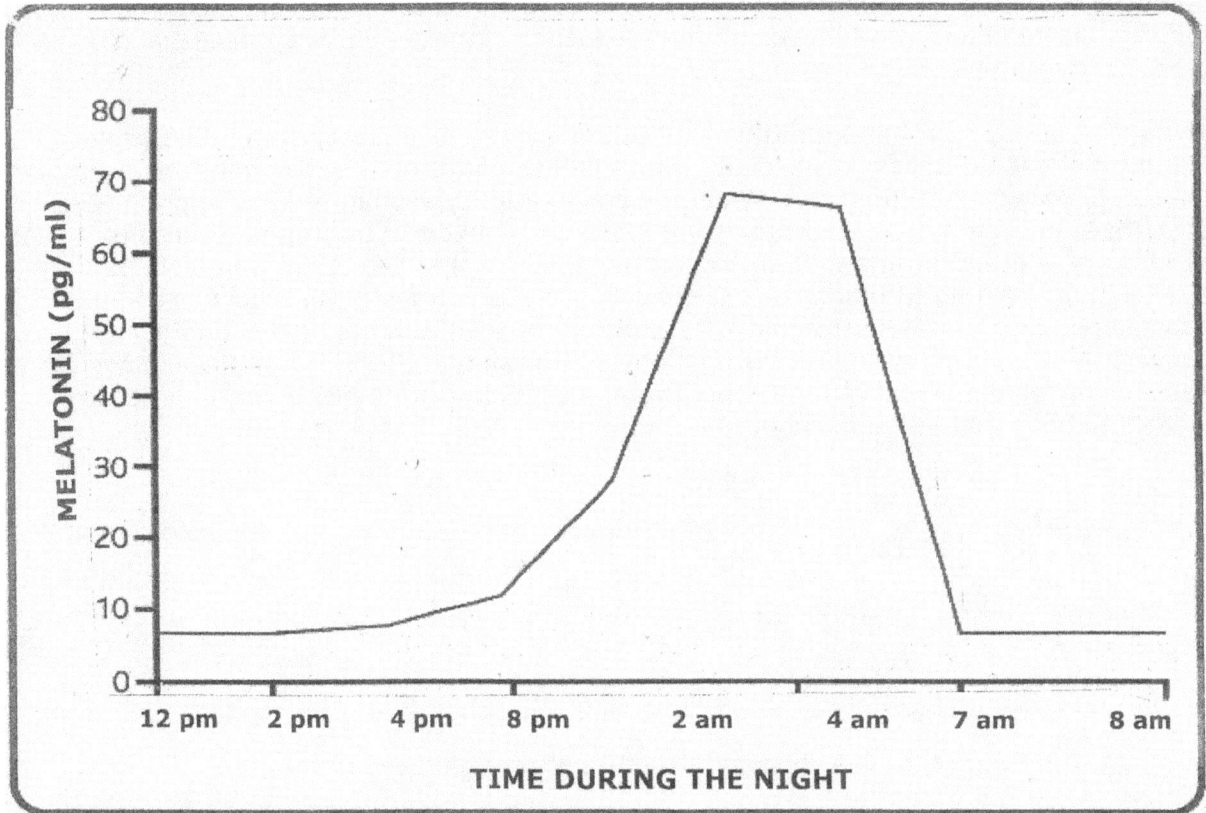

Figure 5.6 The rise and fall of melatonin level during a typical day.

Blood level of melatonin is expressed in picograms per milliliter of blood (pg/ml).

1 milligram = 1,000,000,000 picograms = 10^9 picograms
1 gram   = 1,000,000,000,000 picograms = 10^{12} picograms
1 kilogram = 1,000,000,000,000,000 picograms = 10^{15} picograms

Table 5.1 The rise and fall of melatonin level during a typical day.

TIME	MELATONIN LEVEL
Between 2 pm and 8 pm	Melatinine level begins to rise slightly.
Between 8 pm and 2 am	Melatonin level rises sharply.
Between 2 am and 4 am	Melatonin level reaches its peak level (70 pg/ml).
At 4 am	Melatonin level begins to fall sharply.
At 7 am	Melatonin level drops to its lowest level (about 5 pg/ml).
During the day	Melatonin activity is shut down as the pineal gland does not secrete.

DAYLIGHT ACTIVATES SEROTONIN AND MOONLIGHT STIMULATES MELATONIN

Serotonin and melatonin have opposite functions. The sunshine during the day passes through the retinas of our eyes, and activates and promotes serotonin production, which induces us the joyous feeling. As the day fades away, moonlight stimulates the pineal gland to manufacture and secrete melatonin and tells us it is time to sleep. Daylight has the inhibition effect on melatonin production where as moonlight has stimulation effect.

If the pineal gland situated in your brain secretes normal levels of melatonin during the night, you don't need to supplement melatonin. Artificial melatonin, available as pills or liquid drops in health food stores, is unnecessary. The pineal gland is capable to manufacture and secrete as much melatonin as your body needs to fall asleep and maintain sleep as long as you know how to reset your master biological clock. By living under bright light during the day and by living in the dark during the night, you can reset your master biological clock in a couple of days. Refer to the main article of this course to learn how to reset your master biological clock.

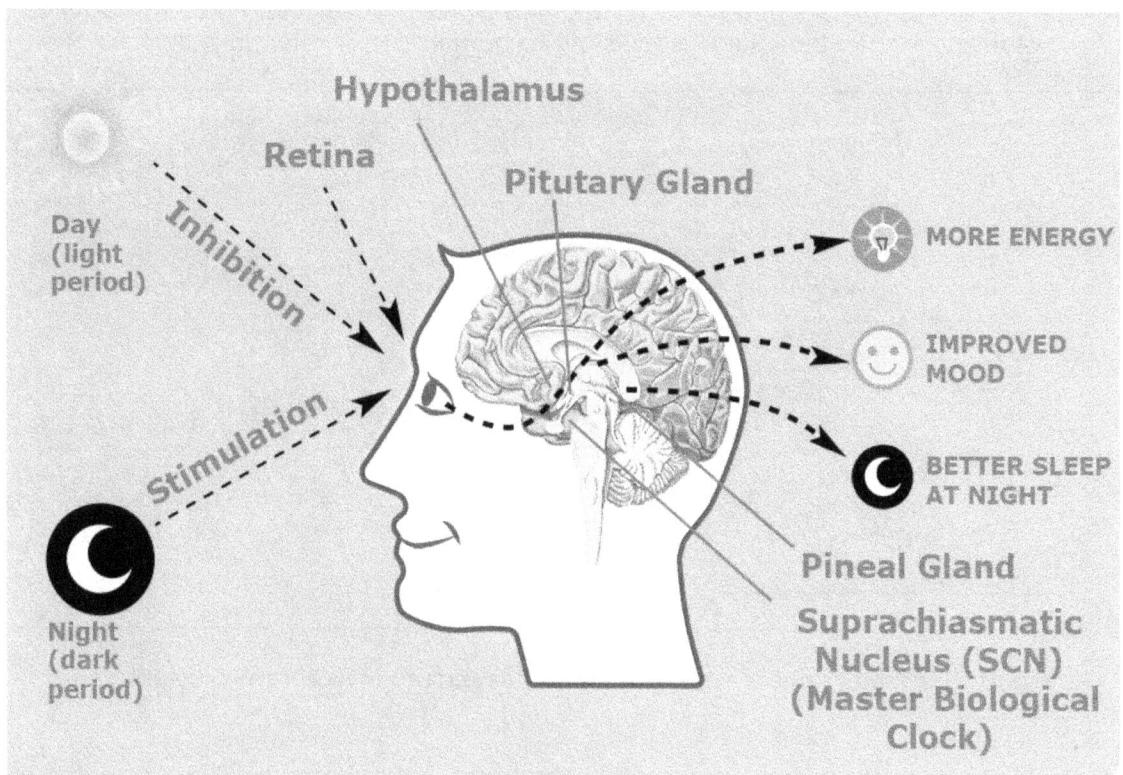

Figure 5.7 Sunlight promotes serotonin production and moonlight promotes melatonin.

BLUE LIGHT AT NIGHT IS HARMFUL AND ADVERSELY AFFECTS THE CIRCADIAN RHYTHM, MORE SPECIFICALLY THE SLEEP-WAKE CYCLE

Sir Isaac Newton (1642-1727) is an English mathematician, an influential scientist, astronomer and physicist. In 1672, he published a series of experiments, demonstrating that white light from the sun or the sunlight is a mixture of the 7 colors of a rainbow "RED, ORANGE, YELLOW, GREEN, BLUE, INDIGO and VIOLET".

WHY IS THE SKY BLUE? [21] Sir Isaac Newton through conducting experiments proved that when white light shines through a glass prism, the light is separated into 7 different colors of the rainbow, forming a spectrum as shown in the picture below. All light is made up of electromagnetic particles that travel in waves. Blue light has shorter wavelength, high frequency and high energy compared to green, yellow, orange and red light. When sunlight travels through the Earth's atmosphere, its blue light is scattered in all directions by all tiny particles and gases present in the air. Blue-colored light is scattered in all directions faster than other colors because it travels in shorter and smaller waves with high energy. This is why we find that the **"SKY IS BLUE"**. Ultraviolet light, with much shorter wavelength than blue light, is invisible to human eye and is more harmful than blue light.

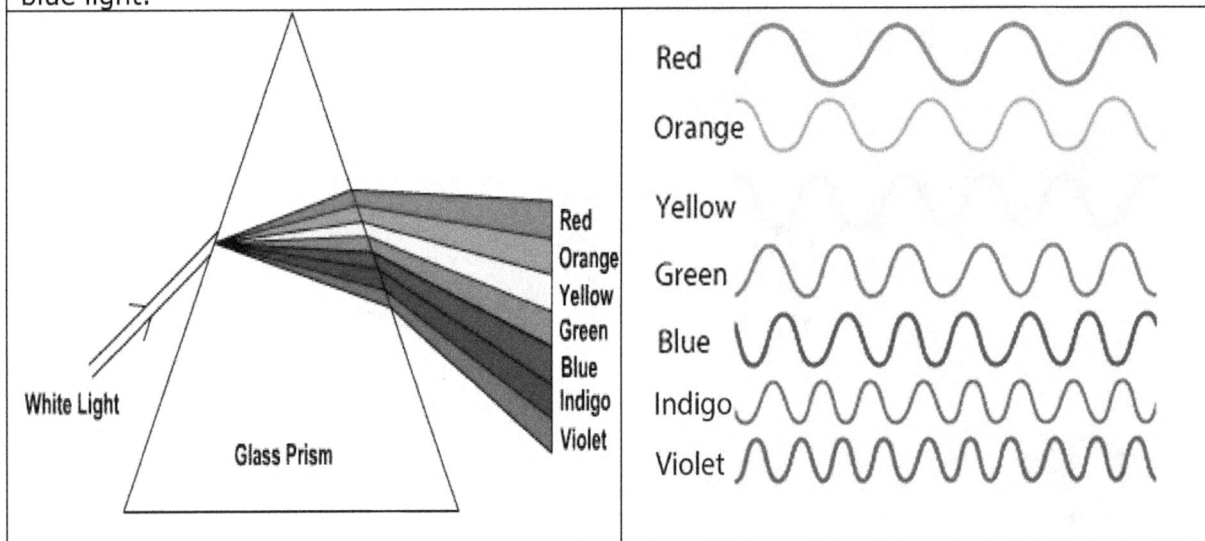

Figure 5.8 White light is separated into a spectrum of 7 different colors.

The frequency of a light wave is expressed in terahertz, abbreviated as THz. The terahertz is a unit of electromagnetic (EM) wave frequency equal to one trillion hertz (10^{12} Hz). The terahertz is used as an indicator of the frequency of infrared (IR), visible, and ultraviolet (UV) radiation. The frequency and wavelength of different kinds of light are shown in the following table. The wavelength of the light shortens as the frequency increases. That means the higher energy lights such as blue light and ultraviolet light, by having shorter wavelengths and higher frequencies are harmful to the human eye. Beware of blue light and ultraviolet light!

Table 5.2 Frequencies and wavelengths of all colors of light. [22]

Color of Light	Energy Level	Frequency (Terahertz, THz)	Wavelength (Nanometers)
Infrared	Lowest	< 300	> 1000
Red		430-480	700-635
Orange		480-510	635-590
Yellow		510-540	590-560
Green	Medium	540-580	560-520
Cyan/Indigo		580-610	520-490
Blue		610-670	490-450
Violet/Purple		670-750	450-400
Ultraviolet	Highest	1000	300
Far Ultraviolet	Highest	> 1500	< 200

As shown in the picture below, blue light has shorter wavelength, high frequency and high energy compared to Green, Yellow, Orange and Red Lights. So you should avoid exposing yourself to blue light.

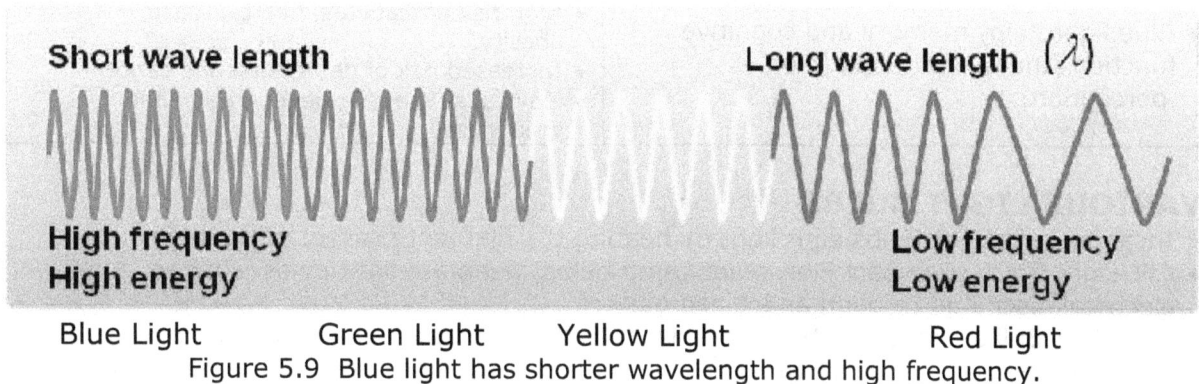

Figure 5.9 Blue light has shorter wavelength and high frequency.

SOURCES OF BLUE LIGHT
Blue Light is also called HEV Light (High-Energy Visible Light).
OUTDOOR SOURCE OF BLUE LIGHT (NATURAL): Sunlight

INDOOR SOURCES OF BLUE LIGHT (ARTIFICIAL):
Digital Flat Screens of TVs, Computers, Laptops or Notebooks, Smart Phones, Electronic Devices, Florescent Lighting, and LED (Light-Emitting Diode) Lighting.

The amount of blue light emitted by these indoors gadget per hour is only a tiny fraction of the blue light being emitted by sunshine when you go out and get exposed to the sun outdoors. But the number of hours a person is exposed to bright lights at nighttime by staying in proximity to electronic screens is significantly high compared to the number of hours one is exposed to the sun. This kind of lifestyle therefore causes eyestrain, macular degeneration, cataracts, snow blindness, a pinguecula, pterygium, and even cancer. [23]

Too much blue light exposure at nighttime more importantly disrupts the melatonin production, and affects a person's sleep-wake cycle thereby causing insomnia or sleeplessness.

As the blue light has visible light with shorter wavelength and high energy, it flickers more easily than the lights with a longer wavelength and low energy. This flickering creates a glare that can reduce visual contrast and adversely affect the sharpness and clarity, thereby causing eyestrain, headaches, and both physical and metal fatigue after sitting long hours in front of the screen of the computer and other electronics. [24]

ADVANTAGES & DISADVANTAGES OF BLUE LIGHT

Blue light has both advantages and disadvantages: [24]

Table 5.3 Adavantages and disadvantages of blue light.

ADVANTAGES OF BLUE LIGHT Limited Blue Light Exposure Is Good!	DISADVANTAGES OF BLUE LIGHT Overexposure to Blue Light Is Harmful!
♦ Helps regulate circadian rhythms, and the body's natural sleep-wake cycle. ♦ Blue light improves mood & alertness. ♦ Blue light helps memory and cognitive function (the mental process of perception).	♦ Disrupt circadian rhythm, and sleep-wake cycle. ♦ Causes eyestrain, blurred vision, dry & irritated eyes, headaches, neck pain, back pain. ♦ High risk of diabetes, heart disease, obesity. ♦ Increased risk of depression and cancer ♦ May cause macular degeneration and vision loss.

VARIOUS LIGHT BULBS [25]

♦ Incandescent Light Bulbs emit light by heating the filament present in the bulb.
♦ CFL Light Bulbs (Compact Florescent Lamp bulbs) generate light by sending an electrical discharge through an ionized gas.
♦ LED Light Bulbs (Light-Emitting Diode Light Bulbs) are assembled into a lamp for use in lighting fixtures. LED lamps have a lifespan and electrical efficiency, which are several times greater than incandescent lamps, and are significantly more efficient than most fluorescent lamps.

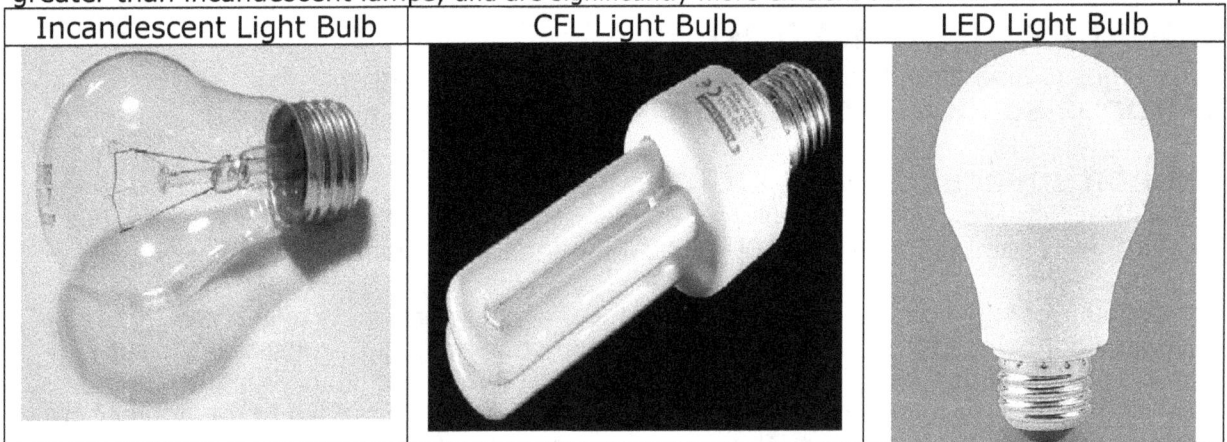

Incandescent Light Bulb	CFL Light Bulb	LED Light Bulb

Figure 5.10 Various light bulbs (Incandescent, CFL & LED).

In 1981, Dr. Charles Czeisler of Harvard Medical School showed that daylight keeps a person's internal biological clock aligned with the environment. While blue light during the daytime has health benefits, the exposure to blue light during the nighttime adversely affects the circadian rhythms, more specifically the sleep-wake cycle. Those who work in the night shifts are more likely to experience disruptive sleep-wake cycle. The circadian rhythm disorder could ultimately lead to diabetes, heart disease, obesity, insomnia and cancer. [26]

In a study conducted at Harvard University, the researchers assigned night work by sitting under bright lights to a group of 10 people, and noticed that their circadian rhythms shifted, their blood sugar levels increased, making them pre-diabetic, and their leptin levels (leptin is a hormone that makes the people feel full after a meal) went down. [26]

In another study conducted at Harvard University, the researchers conducted an experiment in which (i) a group of people were exposed to blue light for 6.5 hours at night, and (ii) another group of people were exposed to green light for 6.5 hours at night. They found that the melatonin levels of the first group who were exposed to blue light suppressed twice and circadian rhythm was shifted by 3 hours, compared to the second group who were exposed to green light and whose circadian rhythm shifted by only 1.5 hours. Which means exposing to blue light at night for prolonged hours is harmful and could shift circadian rhythms. [26]

A researcher Richard Hansler at John Carroll University in Cleveland says that, though all light bulbs produce blue light, the ordinary Incandescent Light Bulbs produce less blue light than the CFL Light Bulbs and LED Light Bulbs. [26]

In another study conducted at the University of Toronto, the researchers conducted an experiment (i) by exposing a group of people to indoor bright lights by wearing the blue-light blocking glasses, and (ii) by exposing another group of people to indoor dim lights. And then they monitored the melatonin levels of both groups by collecting the saliva/blood samples at different intervals of time. They found that the melatonin levels were almost the same in both groups. This study suggests that blue light is the melatonin suppressor, and by wearing the blue-light blocking glasses, it is possible to improve your melatonin levels even if you are working late in the night exposing yourself to bright lights.

An Article Published in the Endocrine Society's Journal of Clinical Endocrinology & Metabolism Concluded the Following: When compared with dim light, exposure to room light during the night suppressed melatonin levels by around 85 percent in trials. [27]

RECOMMENDATIONS FOR BETTER SLEEP
The Harvard Medical School in a Harvard Medical Letter posted the following recommendations for the better sleep: [25, 26, 27]
♦ Use DIM lights as night lights. Red lights (with lowest energy and highest wavelength) have least power to suppress the melatonin level and to shift circadian rhythms.
So use red lights if possible.
♦ Avoid working under bright lights beginning two to three hours before going to bed.
♦ If you work a night shift and/or use electronic devices (computer monitors, laptops, notebooks or other) a lot at night by looking into the electronic screens, consider wearing blue-light blocking glasses.
♦ Expose yourself to lots of sunshine or bright lights during the day, which would boost your mood and alertness during the daytime, and improve your ability to fall asleep easily during the nighttime.

CIRCADIAN RHYTHM DISORDER

If you live carefully following the cues (cue=an indirect suggestion perceived by your body) of your body, your circadian rhythm will remain balanced. [28, 29, 30]

For example, if your body (your master biological clock) tells you to go to bed at 10 pm, and if you follow that indirect suggestion carefully by practicing self-discipline, your circadian rhythm will remain balanced. And if you stay focused on your computer, work till late at night, and do not make the habit of going to bed at 10 pm continuously for several months, then there is a good chance your master biological clock and therefore your circadian rhythm will get disturbed and unbalanced. As a result, you could develop circadian rhythm disorder, and eventually insomnia. When the normal sleep pattern is disturbed and the master biological clock is shifted, a patient is unable to go to sleep, and remain asleep during the regular nighttime hours. If this happens the patient develops one or more of the following circadian rhythm disorders:

1. Jet Lag

When a person travels by plane suddenly to a new intercontinental time zone, which is a few hours to many hours ahead or behind the local time where he/she lives, the person is at a risk of developing the circadian rhythm disorder called "Jet Lag". For example if an American traveler who lives in Los Angeles travels to China where the time is 12 to 14 hours ahead of Los Angeles, he/she is bound to experience "Jet Lag". Most people get used to the new location within a few days. Though Jet Lag is a temporary disorder, it could become a serious disorder if the person's job demands frequent travel between different time zones. For elderly people, it would be much more difficult to adapt to a new time zone, and Jet Lag could be a serious problem.

2. Shift Work Sleep Disorder

If a person works in irregular shifts till late in the night, and changes his/her sleep schedule significantly without sleeping during the regular nighttime hours, the person could develop sleeplessness, fatigue and exhaustion. The person's master biological clock shifts and the person could develop another kind of circadian sleep disorder called "Shift Work Sleep Disorder."

3. Non-24-Hour Sleep-Wake Syndrome/Free Running Disorder

Blind people most commonly develop this Non-24-Hour Sleep-Wake Syndrome because the retinas of the eyes, by not functioning properly, become unable to sense light or darkness correctly and fail to send accurate signals to the suprachiasmatic nucleus (SCN) or the master biological clock, resulting in the failure to produce melatonin appropriately in the nighttime. As a result, the sleep-wake cycle of blind people keeps shifting over and over again indefinitely. It was reported that more than half of blind people suffer from this kind of circadian rhythm disorder.

4. Delayed Sleep-Wake Phase

In this kind of sleep disorder, a person is unable to go to bed during regular nighttime hours, but goes to bed several hours later, spending time watching TV or doing some other activity, but staying awake. The pineal gland of a person with this kind of sleep disorder produces melatonin 2 or more hours later. So, the person even wakes up several hours later in the morning too. People with this kind of sleep disorder could even miss their work schedule by going to work several hours late.

5. Advanced Sleep-Wake Phase

In this kind of sleep disorder, a person is tempted to go to bed several hours before the regular hours, advancing himself/herself several hours of the sleep-wake cycle. The pineal gland of a person with this kind of sleep disorder produces melatonin prematurely 2 or more hours in advance. This person goes to bed earlier than the normal hours of the nighttime and wakes up in the morning several hours earlier too. Most people with this sleep disorder complain of early-morning insomnia and day-time sleepiness.

6. Irregular Sleep-Wake Rhythm

People with this kind of sleep disorder do not fit into the descriptions of any other sleep disorder as explained above. Instead, they experience the sleep-wake cycle throughout the day and throughout the night. They keep taking short naps throughout the day (24 hours). They do not have any definite schedule for sleep and to stay awake, indicating irregular sleep-wake cycle. People with mental disorders such as dementia, brain damage and mental retardation usually experience this kind of circadian rhythm disorder.

TREATMENT FOR CIRCADIAN RHYTHM DISORDER

Please refer to Chapter 1 of this book, and please follow the 24 instructions outlined in the main article of REVERSING INSOMNIA course.

DURING THE DAY	DURING THE NIGHT
◉ DURING THE DAY, YOU ESSENTIALLY LIVE UNDER SUNLIGHT OR BRIGHT LIGHTS WHENEVER YOU ARE OUTDOORS OR UNDER BRIGHT LIGHTS WHENEVER YOU ARE INDOORS.	◉ DURING THE NIGHT, YOU ESSENTIALLY LIVE IN THE DARK BY STAYING AT HOME (ALWAYS STAY INDOORS) AND DO NOT GO OUT AND DO NOT EXPOSE YOURSELF TO BRIGHT LIGHTS.
◉ BY DOING SO, YOU WOULD LET YOUR BRAIN KNOW EXACTLY WHICH HOURS ARE THE DAY (For example 6 am to 6 pm or 7 am to 7 pm or 8 am to 8 pm). Each person is different so you can choose your DAY hours.	◉ BY DOING SO, YOU WOULD LET YOUR BRAIN KNOW EXACTLY WHICH HOURS ARE THE NIGHT (For example 6 pm to 6 am or 7 pm to 7 am or 8 pm to 8 am). Each person is different so you can choose your NIGHT hours.

By living under sunlight or bright lights during the day, and by living strictly in the dark during the night, without exposure to bright lights, it is possible to reverse circadian rhythm disorder. This is the fundamental principle based on which the method of reversing insomnia has been derived and outlined in this book in Chapter 1.

REFERENCES

1. Circadian Rhythm (from Wikipedia).
https://en.wikipedia.org/wiki/Circadian_rhythm

2. How to Get Better Sleep: The Beginner's Guide to Overcoming Sleep Deprivation by James Clear at Better Sleep. a. http://jamesclear.com/better-sleep
b. http://jamesclear.com/articles

3. What is Earth's location in space?
http://coolcosmos.ipac.caltech.edu/ask/62-What-is-Earth-s-location-in-space-

4. Kepler's Universe: More Planets in Our Galaxy Than Stars, by Nancy Atkinson, Article Updated: Jan 13, 2016.
https://www.universetoday.com/109551/keplers-universe-more-planets-in-our-galaxy-than-stars/

5. Earth's Rotation.
https://en.wikipedia.org/wiki/Earth%27s_rotation

6. How long does the Earth take to go around the Sun and what causes the seasons? September 15, 2010.
https://maas.museum/observations/2010/09/15/how-long-does-the-earth-take-to-go-around-the-sun-and-what-causes-the-seasons/

7. Circadian Rhythms Fact Sheet, National Institute of General Medical Sciences.
https://www.nigms.nih.gov/education/pages/Factsheet_CircadianRhythms.aspx

8. Master Body Clock and Circadian Rhythms.
http://www.non-24.com/circadian-rhythms.php

9. Cool facts about your biological clock by Eleanor Imster, November 3, 2014.
http://earthsky.org/human-world/cool-facts-about-your-biological-clock

10. Pineal Gland, Functions, Melatonin & Circadian rhythm.
http://study.com/academy/lesson/pineal-gland-functions-melatonin-circadian-rhythm.html

11. Sleep Series – Part 3: Serotonin, Melatonin, and your Circadian Rhythm by Graham Ballachey, May 13, 2014.
http://sustainablebalance.ca/serotonin-melatonin-and-your-circadian-rhythm/

12. Serotonin: Facts, What Does Serotonin Do? by James Mcintosh, Last updated Fri 29 April 2016.
https://www.medicalnewstoday.com/kc/serotonin-facts-232248

13. Boosting Your Serotonin Activity, 4 ways to boost your serotonin! by Alex Korb, PhD, Posted Nov 17, 2011.
https://www.psychologytoday.com/blog/prefrontal-nudity/201111/boosting-your-serotonin-activity

14. The Pineal Gland and Melatonin, Author: R. Bowen, March 17, 2003.
http://www.vivo.colostate.edu/hbooks/pathphys/endocrine/otherendo/pineal.html

15. Serotonin Vs. Melatonin, by Clay McNight, April 23, 2015.
http://www.livestrong.com/article/336314-serotonin-vs-melatonin/

16. Hormones, Neurotransmitters and SAD (Seasonal Affective Disorder).
http://www.educationdx.com/seasonal-affective-hormones.html

17. Melatonin the "light of night" in human biology and adolescent idiopathic scoliosis, Theodoros B Grivas and Olga D Savvidou.
https://www.ncbi.nlm.nih.gov/pmc/articles/PMC1855314/

18. Book: Alternative Medicine Magazine's Definitive Guide to Sleep Disorders: 7 Smart Ways to Help You Get a Good Night's Rest Kindle Edition by Herbert Ross and Keri Brenner.

19. Three Simple Ways That I Optimize My Sleep by Brian Martinek.
https://brianmartinek.com/three-simple-ways-that-i-optimize-my-sleep/

20. Circadian Rhythms: How Sleep Works
https://www.howsleepworks.com/how_circadian.html

21. Why Sky is Blue?, NASA Space Place, Explore Earth and Space.
https://spaceplace.nasa.gov/blue-sky/en/

22. Color, from Wikipedia.
https://en.wikipedia.org/wiki/Color

23. Blue Light: It's Both Bad And Good For You, by Gary Heiting, OD.
http://www.allaboutvision.com/cvs/blue-light.htm

24. Blue Light Exposed.
http://www.bluelightexposed.com/#where-is-the-increased-exposure-to-blue-light-coming-from
http://www.bluelightexposed.com/#where-is-blue-light-found

25. Choosing the right light bulbs for your home.
https://sleep.org/articles/choosing-lightbulbs/

26. Blue Light Has a Dark Side, exposure to blue light at night, emitted by electronics and energy-efficient lightbulbs, harmful to your health, Published: May, 2012, Updated on September 2, 2015.
http://www.health.harvard.edu/staying-healthy/blue-light-has-a-dark-side

27. How Blue LEDs Effect Sleep by Alina Bradford, Live Science Contributor, Feb 26, 2016.
http://www.livescience.com/53874-blue-light-sleep.html

28. Circadian Rhythm and Your Body Clock: Understanding your body's internal clock—or circadian rhythm—is the first step to better sleep.
https://sleep.org/articles/circadian-rhythm-body-clock/

29. 6 Circadian Rhythm Sleep Disorders that May Be Disrupting Your Sleep, Posted by Kevin Phillips on Nov 17, 2014.
http://www.alaskasleep.com/blog/circadian-rhythm-sleep-disorders-disrupting-your-sleep

30. Circadian Rhythm Sleep-Wake Disorders.
http://www.sleepeducation.org/sleep-disorders-by-category/circadian-rhythm-disorders

CHAPTER 6: REM STAGE OF SLEEP

TABLE OF CONTENTS

HUMAN SLEEP TAKES PLACE IN 5 STAGES

Sleep researchers discovered the REM sleep (REM = Rapid Eye Movement Sleep) in 1953.[1] REM stage of sleep is primarily characterized by movements of the eyes and is the fifth stage of sleep.

Until 1953, humans thought that the brain is dormant or stagnant while sleeping, but the opposite is true as the brain is very active while sleeping. Sleep helps our body and brain develop and grow stronger. We need to sleep so that we remember what we learn in our lives, pay attention to the things we have done and are about to do, concentrate or focus on our tasks and ideas, solve problems and plan an agenda of what to do in the future with both short and long-term goals. [2]

Table 6.1 Human sleep takes place in 5 stages.

The HUMAN SLEEP takes place in cycles and within each cycle, there are 5 stages. The first 4 stages are called non-REM stages. The 5th stage is called the REM stage of sleep. We spend almost 50% of our total sleep time in STAGE 2 sleep, about 20% in REM sleep, and the remaining 30% in the other stages. Infants, by contrast, spend about half of their sleep time in REM sleep. For a healthy person, a complete sleep cycle (all 5 stages) takes 90 to 110 minutes on an average, depending on the person and the condition of health. [2]	
STAGE 1 Non-REM Stage	Beta State of Mind, Brain Wave Frequency = 14-40 CPS or Htzs. Brain waves have the highest frequency & lowest amplitude, the person is awake.
STAGE 2 Non-REM Stage	Alpha State of Mind, Brain Wave Frequency = 7-14 CPS or Htzs. Brain waves have lower frequency & higher amplitude. Relaxed and day-dreaming state of mind, light sleep, meditation, intuition, a person becomes increasingly sleepy. Heart rate & body temp drop.
STAGE 3 Non-REM Stage	Theta State of Mind, Brain Wave Frequency = 4-7 CPS or Htzs. Metabolic rate is slowest and growth hormones are produced. Brain waves have much lower frequency and much higher amplitude. Highly meditative and much deeper stage of sleep. Body strengthens its immune system, repairs and regrows muscles and tissues, and builds bone structures.
STAGE 4 Non-REM Stage	Delta State of Mind, Brain Wave Frequency = 0.1-4 CPS or Htzs. Brain waves have much lower frequency and much higher amplitude. The body is asleep, mind is awake and almost unconscious. Deepest sleep, meditative & lazy brain waves; about an hour after the person falls asleep. Talking and walking in the sleep, bed-wetting occurs but not remembered. Metabolic rate is slowest and growth hormones are produced. Body temperature and blood pressure further drops.
STAGE 5 REM STAGE OR DREAM STAGE	**REM (Rapid Eye Movement) Stage/Dream Stage**: Brain waves exhibit the combined effect of theta, alpha and beta, and desynchronous waves. [3, 4] ♦ Paradoxical sleep occurs, as the body's arms, legs and muscles become relaxed and paralyzed, and the brain is very active, the eyes move rapidly, and REM sleep occurs. ♦ The sleeper's legs, face and fingers twitch. The breathing is shallow. ♦ The heart rate, blood pressure and body temperature increase. ♦ Intense dreaming with vivid visual imagery, sounds, smells etc. is often reported. ♦ A lot of energy is provided to the brain and body so you burn 3 times more calories during REM sleep.

When a healthy person sleeps for 8 to 9 hours, there would be 5 to 6 cycles of sleep, going through the REM stage 5 to 6 times each night. The first sleep cycle contains relatively short REM periods and long periods of deep sleep. The first REM sleep period usually occurs for about 70 to 90 minutes. As the night progresses, REM sleep periods increase in length, while deep sleep decreases as shown in the diagram below. By morning, people spend nearly all their sleep time in stages 1, 2 and REM. [2]

During the REM Stage of Sleep (during the Dream Stage), the brain waves exhibit the combined effect of beta, alpha and theta, and desynchronous waves. [3, 4]

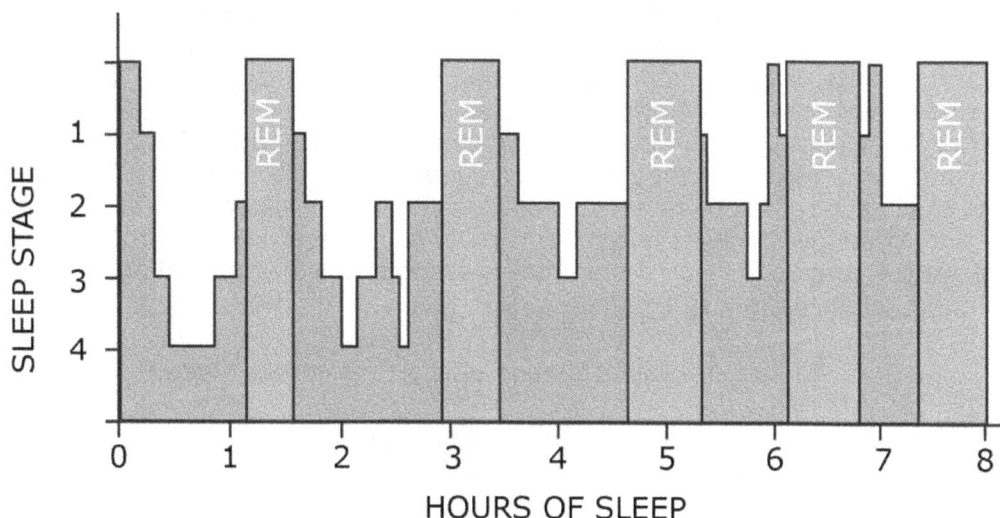

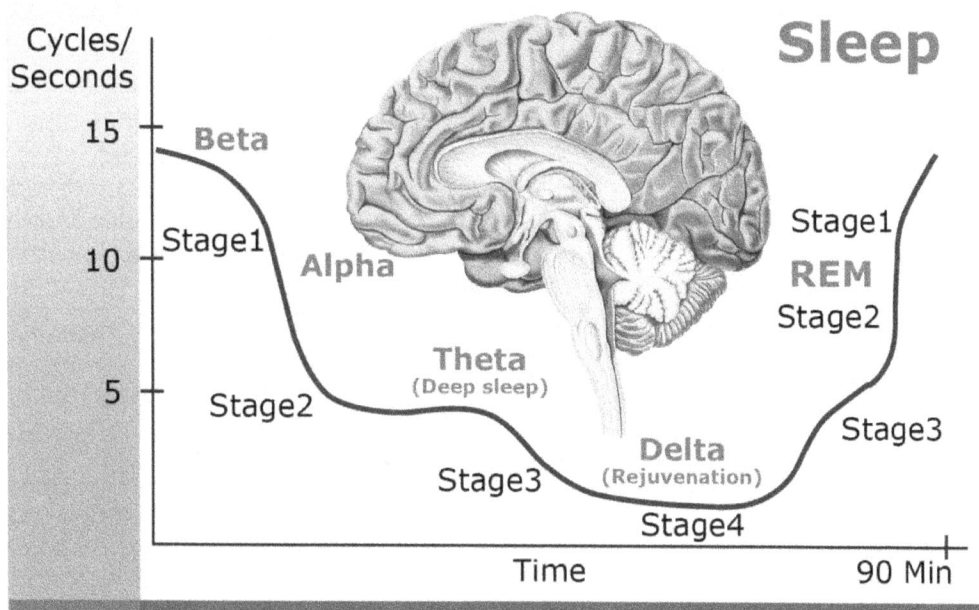

Figure 6.1 REM stage period gradually increases as the night progresses.

The Sleep, Brain Wave Frequencies and States of Mind [5, 6]

In neuroscience, there are five states of mind namely Beta, Alpha, Theta, Delta and the lesser known state of mind Gamma. When a person relaxes and falls asleep, the brain wave frequencies slow down with increased amplitude, and the calm consciousness switches from the beta state, which is the normal waking state to the deeper states of consciousness such as Alpha, Theta or Delta. The brain wave frequencies can be monitored in a sleep lab by conducting the EEG test (Electroencephalography) on the patient, as shown in the diagram below. When a person's consciousness reaches the Theta state during sleep, the person starts entering the dream state, which is called the REM stage of sleep (During the REM stage of sleep, the consciousness switches back to both Alpha and Beta states, as the brain becomes more and more active). Theta state is also called the realm of the subconscious mind. More than 90% of your mind is subconscious mind in which all your life story of this life, all the past lives and all memories are stored and readily available and accessible. When the consciousness switches to a much deeper state of mind, called Delta state, the person becomes unconscious in the sleep (body sleeps but mind is awake). This is the gateway to the super-conscious mind, collective unconscious, also called the universal mind or God's mind whereby the divine information could be received which otherwise would be unavailable at the conscious level. Delta state is associated with the healing, guidance to good health, abundance, prosperity, inner peace, love and spiritual growth. [5]

Table 6.2 Brain frequencies chart during the sleep.

State of Mind	Brainwave Frequency (CPS/Hertz)	Associated With
Beta Waves — Frequency: 12 to 30 Hz	12 – 30	Normal waking state, alertness, focus, cognition, working all 5 senses, perception of time and space.
Alpha Waves — Frequency: 7.5 to 12 Hz	7 – 12	Deep relaxation, light sleep with eyes closed, meditation, visualization, creativity, intuition and super learning. No time and space limitation.
Theta Waves — Frequency: 4 to 7.5 Hz	4 – 7.5	Deeper sleep, usually light sleep, deeper meditation, intuition, memory, vivid visual imagery, REM state.
Delta Waves — Frequency: up to 4 Hz	0.1 – 4	Much Deeper sleep, dreamless state, almost unconscious, automatic self-healing, imune system functioning, (body asleep, mind awake).

INFLUENCE OF SLEEP ON THE HUNGER HORMONES "LEPTIN AND GHRELIN" AND BODY WEIGHT [7, 8, 9]

LEPTIN: The name leptin is derived from the Greek word 'leptos' meaning thin. It is sometimes referred to as the 'Fat Controller'. Leptin is a hormone secreted from fat cells, in the adipose tissue, that helps to regulate body weight. Leptin levels give signals to the brain whenever you have eaten enough to induce satiety or a feeling of fullness, when it is time to burn calories and when it is time to create energy for your survival. Leptin also triggers messages between the hypothalamus and thyroid gland which controls the storage and adequate use of the energy for the body's survival whenever needed.

The amount of leptin of a person is directly related to the amount of body fat. Obese people have more leptin and slim people have less leptin. When a person is obese, the brain does not respond to leptin and the person does not feel full (no feeling of satiation), developing leptin resistance. So an obese person eats even more and gains more weight. The hormone leptin is a chemical substance that regulates appetite, metabolism and calorie burning. During sleep, leptin levels increase sending the brain a signal that the energy levels are good and that there is no need to eat food for more energy.

GHRELIN: Ghrelin, also called the 'Growth Hormone', is produced by specialized cells located in the stomach and the pancreas. Ghrelin stimulates hunger. Ghrelin levels increase before meals and decrease after meals, and is regulated in the hypothalamus of the brain. The purpose of ghrelin is basically the exact opposite of leptin.

It tells your brain when you need to eat, when your body should stop burning calories and when it should store energy as fat. Ghrelin plays an important role in hunger and therefore weight gain. If you sleep well, the ghrelin level decreases. If you don't sleep well, the ghrelin level increases, making you feel hungry. So you eat more food and gain weight. And the body stops burning calories because the brain thinks that you would be starving in the near future and signals the thyroid to store fat calories for the future use. As a result, the weight gain continues.

ENOUGH SLEEP: Low ghrelin, high leptin, normal appetite and satisfied after eating.
POOR SLEEP: High ghrelin, low leptin, feels hungry, makes you overeat and gain weight.

Table 6.3 Difference Between hunger hormones ghrelin and leptin.

GHRELIN	LEPTIN
Ghrelin is released from stomach, and when elevated, sends a signal to your brain informing you that you are hungry and it is time to eat. In other words, ghrelin tells your body when to eat. Age, gender, blood glucose level, body weight would all influence the ghrelin levels. Lack of sleep would raise ghrelin levels, leading to overeating.	Leptin is stored and secreted by fat cells, and is considered to be the master regulator of hunger. When you eat a meal, leptin is released from fat cells and send a signal to your brain, informing that you full and stop eating. In other words, leptin tells your body when to stop eating. Lack of sleep would lower leptin levels, leading to overeating.

LEPTIN RESISTANCE CYCLE

Leptin and weight gain work hand in hand. When you overeat and gain weight, the body fat increases creating more fat cells. The increased number of fat cells means the increased leptin levels. The increased fat cells and leptin levels develop leptin resistance, thereby the signal to your brain gets disrupted (you brain fails to tell you that you are full and stop eating). The brain mistakenly senses that your leptin levels are too low, and therefore you overeat, resulting in weight gain. And this cycle of leptin resistance continues unless you take action and control it.

BALANCE BETWEEN GHRELIN AND LEPTIN LEVELS IS ESSENTIAL

In order to break the leptin resistance cycle, you should balance your leptin and ghrelin levels by sleeping well (at least 8 hours per night), by eating healthy and by exercising well every day.

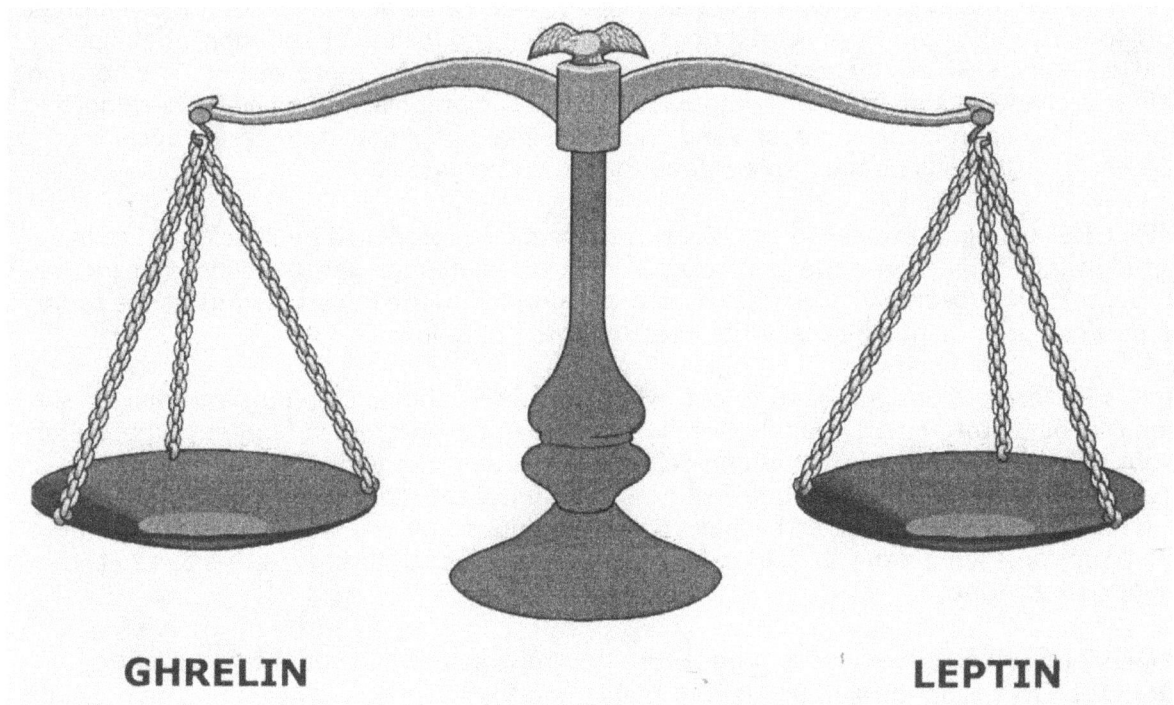

GHRELIN   LEPTIN

Figure 6.2 Balance between ghrelin and leptin levels is essential.

During REM Sleep You Burn 3 Times More Calories [10]

In 2009, a sleep research study conducted in Sao Paulo, Brazil found that while sleeping you burn three times more fat calories than when lying in bed awake. In another study, two groups of sleepers, who were placed on identical diets, participated in a sleep study. The first group of sleepers who slept only 5.5 hours lost the lean muscle as opposed to the second group of sleepers who slept more than 7 hours lost fat. The study concluded that the fat loss of the second group of sleepers took place in the REM stage of sleep.

During the REM stage of sleep, your brain is more active than in any other stage. Some studies showed that the brain in REM stage of sleep is even more active than when the person is awake. This kind of rapid activity during the REM stage of sleep requires fuel, which comes by burning the fat.

IMPORTANCE OF BOTH NON-REM SLEEP AND REM SLEEP

I. Review Posted by Tim Ferriss [11]

Both the Non-REM sleep (Stage 1, Stage 2, Stage 3, Stage 4) and REM sleep (Stage 5) are important. Good sleep is mostly dependent on the ratio of rapid eye movement (REM) to total sleep, not total REM duration alone. The higher the percentage of REM sleep is, the more restful the sleep would be. The higher the REM percentage, the better the recall of skills or data acquired in the previous 24 hours. Higher-percentage REM sleep also correlates to lower average pulse and temperature upon waking. [11]

II. Review Found in the Book of Melinda Boyd, RD and Michele Noonan, PhD, Train Your Brain to Get Thin (Pages 201-207) [12]

RECHARGING YOUR BODY

Non-REM sleep (the first four stages of sleep of a cycle) is needed to recharge your body. In the slow-wave or deep, restorative phases (that is the non-REM stages), the emphasis is on recharging your body, which is necessary to allow it to be restored and ready for the next day. This slow-wave sleep is also what sets the stage for REM sleep, which is needed to recharge your brain.

RECHARGING YOUR BRAIN

REM sleep (the fifth stage of the sleep cycle) is needed to recharge your brain. Once you enter into the REM phase, the focus moves from the body onto your brain. Your breathing becomes shallow, muscle activity slows down, and your heart rate and blood pressure increase, all in an effort to allow your brain to be front and center and a chance to recharge. It is important to have REM sleep because it is essential to learning and memory, both of which can help in changing your habits to healthier ones. Rockefeller University researchers found that in rats those brain cells were activated during the awake time, and also seem to be reactivated during the REM sleep, and this activity can help us better remember what we learned earlier that day.

Your brain does the following during REM sleep:

a. Consolidates and processes the information from everything you have learned throughout the day.
b. Forms neuronal connections that will strengthen your newly-made memories.
c. Replenishes neurotransmitters, including serotonin and dopamine, which are integral to helping all parts of the brain to work to their maximum potential.

Moreover, sleep is known to increase brain plasticity, which is important for helping you continue on learning as you get older.

THE IMPORTANCE OF REM SLEEP

Lack of REM sleep appears to affect our ability to concentrate and remember things. When allowed to sleep uninterrupted, subjects experience REM rebound. That is, they spend twice as much time in REM sleep as normal to make up for the REM sleep lost. This indicates that REM sleep is vital for our survival.

GET THE SLEEP YOU NEED TO GET THIN

It is important to nature deep restoration in both slow-wave sleep and REM sleep (dreaming) because both kind of sleeping stages play a critical role in allowing your brain to properly process, retain and integrate what has happened, what you have done and what you have learned when you were in the preceding wake state.

Allowing yourself to get the right amount of sleep will benefit your brain tremendously, allowing you to keep your brain pliable and functioning at its highest potential. In order to really get the sleep that you need to benefit your brain (and your body), you will need to stay away from things that interfere with your ability to fall asleep and to stay asleep.

Here are the tips you could practice in order to improve your overall quality of sleep:

TIPS FOR BETTER SLEEP

1. Relaxation is critical to helping you to get a good night's sleep. Exercise during the day several hours prior to going to bed. Avoid exercising within 2 hours of heading to bed.

2. Avoid alcohol consumption as it directly affects and reduces the duration of the REM sleep.

3. Eat light in the evening. If you eat a heavy meal, your digestive system would take long hours to work and could interfere with your sleep.

4. Eat smaller portions more frequently and avoid large meals. Practice portion control and lose excess weight if you have any.

5. Stick to a schedule rigorously. Go to bed at the same time and wake up at the same time every day.

6. Create a quiet and comfortable sleep environment in your bedroom. Sleep on a comfortable bed with comfortable pillows. Let there be no noise while you sleep and let the bedroom temperature be between 68°F and 72°F (between 20°C and 22°C).

7. Bring it down a notch. Practice relaxation activities such as stretching, meditation, and breathing before going to bed. Do not work on complicated and highly responsible projects till late night.

8. Avoid caffeine and drink warm milk an hour before going to bed. Milk contains L-tryptophan, an amino acid and precursor of melatonin and serotonin, both of which promote sleep and good mood. Aim for 4 ounces of fat-free or organic skim milk or 1% organic milk if you find that milk does the trick and lulls you off to sleep. (Lull = to cause to fall asleep).

9. Treat your stress. Be in a pleasant and calm mood all the time.
Meditation could improve the state of well-being and relieve the stress.

The trick to getting a good night's sleep may be as simple as reducing stress. Take some time before bed to chill out (chill out = calm down, take everything easy, relax).
The 2007 stress and anxiety disorders study conducted by the Anxiety Disorders Association of America found that, of those adults who suffer from stress-induced sleep difficulties, three-fourths report that the lack of sleep increased their stress levels during the day.
That means there may be more stress later on, which won't help you to break the cycle and

get the sleep that you indeed need in the following night. Cutting back the stress would help you sleep better and allow you to wake up refreshed and ready to face the day with a positive attitude and the readiness to make right choices to keep you healthy.

GOOD SLEEP IS ESSENTIAL FOR YOUR BODY & FOR YOUR BRAIN

A good night's sleep is as good for your body as it is for your brain because:

a. Good sleep promotes your health and well-being.
b. Good sleep allows you to have the time needed for your body and for your brain to restore, repair and regenerate.
c. Good sleep boosts your mood, creates a positive outlook, and increases your energy level throughout the day.
d. Good sleep helps to better handle the normal stress that comes up in everyday life.
e. Good sleep helps your brain to expand and master new life skills.

Neurons in the Human Brain

An axon is a long, slender projection of a nerve cell, or a neuron, that typically conducts electrical impulses away from the neuron's cell body. Axons are also known as nerve fibers. A nerve cell carries information between the brain and other parts of the body. For a long time, neuroscientists believed that the average human brain consists of about 100 billion neurons in the human brain, and in addition the brain has 10 billion of helper cells.

III. Review Posted by James Clear [13]

The sleep cycle is divided into two important parts:
  a. Non-REM Sleep/Slow-Wave Sleep (brain wave frequencies are slow)
  b. REM Sleep (brain wave frequencies are higher, mind is active)
During the slow-wave sleep (alpha, theta and delta states of mind), the body is calm, relaxes, breathing becomes more regular, blood pressure falls, and the brain is quiet and unresponsive to the external environment. During this slow-wave sleep, the pituitary gland releases growth hormones which are necessary for tissue growth and muscle repair, and also the body's immune system is repaired. Slow-wave sleep is being deliberately practiced by professional athletes like Roger Federer (a tennis player) and LeBron James (a basketball player), who sleep some 11 to 12 hours per night. Research showed that the performance of athletes could significantly be improved by allowing them to sleep more hours per night. Slow wave sleep helps athletes recover from physical injuries and to build muscle strength.

During the REM sleep phase, the brain experiences dreams and re-organizes all the information. During this phase, your brain clears out irrelevant information, boosts your memory by connecting the experiences of the last 24 hours to your previous experiences, and facilitates learning and neural growth. Your body temperature rises, your blood pressure increases, and your heart rate speeds up. Despite all of this activity, your body hardly moves. Typically, the REM phase occurs in short bursts, about 3 to 5 times per night. The amount of time you spend in REM sleep phase decreases with age. The older you become, the less REM sleep you get.

If you are not spending enough time in slow wave sleep and REM sleep phase every night, you become sleep deprived, and experience the risk of viral infections, weight gain, diabetes, high blood pressure, heart disease, mental illness and mortality.

Slow wave sleep helps you recover and perform well physically while the REM sleep helps you recover mentally.

IV. Review Posted by Confess-and-Chillax [14]

Researchers have reported that the women who sleep 5 hours or less per night generally weigh more than the women who sleep 7 hours per night. At least 7 hours of sleep is necessary to properly metabolize food, stabilize hormone levels and recharge energy levels, which are all important aspects if you want to lose weight. If you do not sleep enough while trying to lose weight, you are at a higher risk of cardiovascular problems, diabetes, immune system complications and obesity.

NARCOLEPSY EXPLAINED [15, 16, 17]

Statistical data reveal that there are 3 million people worldwide have narcolepsy. In the USA alone, there are about 200,000 people being affected and living with narcolepsy, but not even a quarter of them were diagnosed by their doctors. The prevalence is about 1 per 2,000 people. [15]

Narcolepsy is a neurological sleep disorder caused by the brain dysfunction mechanisms that control sleep-wake cycle. Researchers believe that narcolepsy is caused by the lack of receptors for the neurotransmitter hypocretin, which regulates the sleeping and waking states.

The sudden and uncontrollable sleep episodes may take place at any time, on any day, during any type of activity, even at the workplace or even behind the wheel of a car while driving. Narcolepsy usually begins between the ages of 15 and 25, but a person can experience this sleep disorder at any age. In many cases, narcolepsy is undiagnosed, and therefore untreated. [15]

The Symptoms Include:

(i) Narcolepsy is characterized by excessive short periods of daytime sleepiness and uncontrollable sleep episodes during the daytime at unexpected times.
(ii) People with narcolepsy fall asleep at any time without knowing that they are sleeping.
(iii) People with narcolepsy experience sudden loss of muscle tone while awake whenever they hear a surprising news, or whenever they are upset or becomes angry,
(iv) People with narcolepsy experience vivid hallucinations in sleep, sleep attacks throughout the day accompanied by short periods of REM stage of sleep, sleep paralysis of large muscles during the REM stage of sleep.

NARCOLEPSY AND SLEEP APNEA TOGETHER [17]

Even though the diagnosis for these two sleep disorders "narcolepsy and sleep apnea" is very different, a person may experience both disorders at the same time. By monitoring and understanding the symptoms that a person experiences, it is possible to determine which disorder is more dominant. But what is known to the researchers is that sleep apnea may interrupt with narcolepsy diagnosis. It not only delays the evaluation of narcolepsy but also interrupts treatment initiatives. It is also known that the deployment of CPAP (Continuous Positive Air Pressure) therapy with a narcolepsy patient has no effect on daytime sleepiness, when he or she is also affected by sleep apnea. While the CPAP machine keeps the blood oxygen levels perfectly normal, it does not help the patient to stay awake during the daytime. If a narcolepsy patient is experiencing low blood oxygen levels, he/she must use CPAP therapy even during the day to treat the sleep disorder.

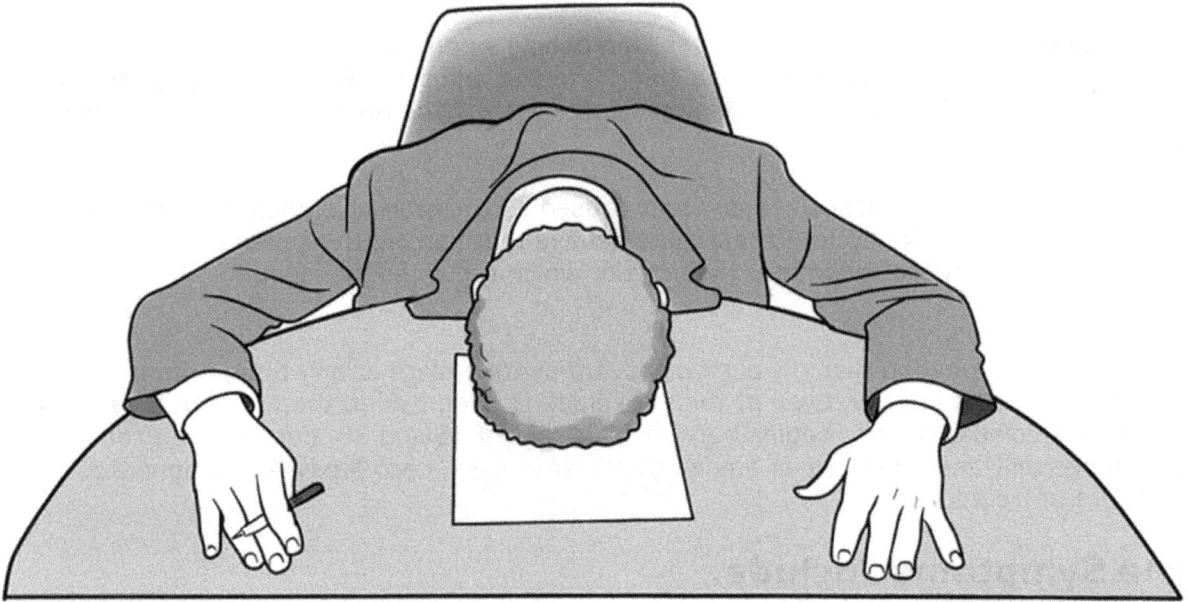

Figure 6.3 A person with narcolepsy fell asleep at work.

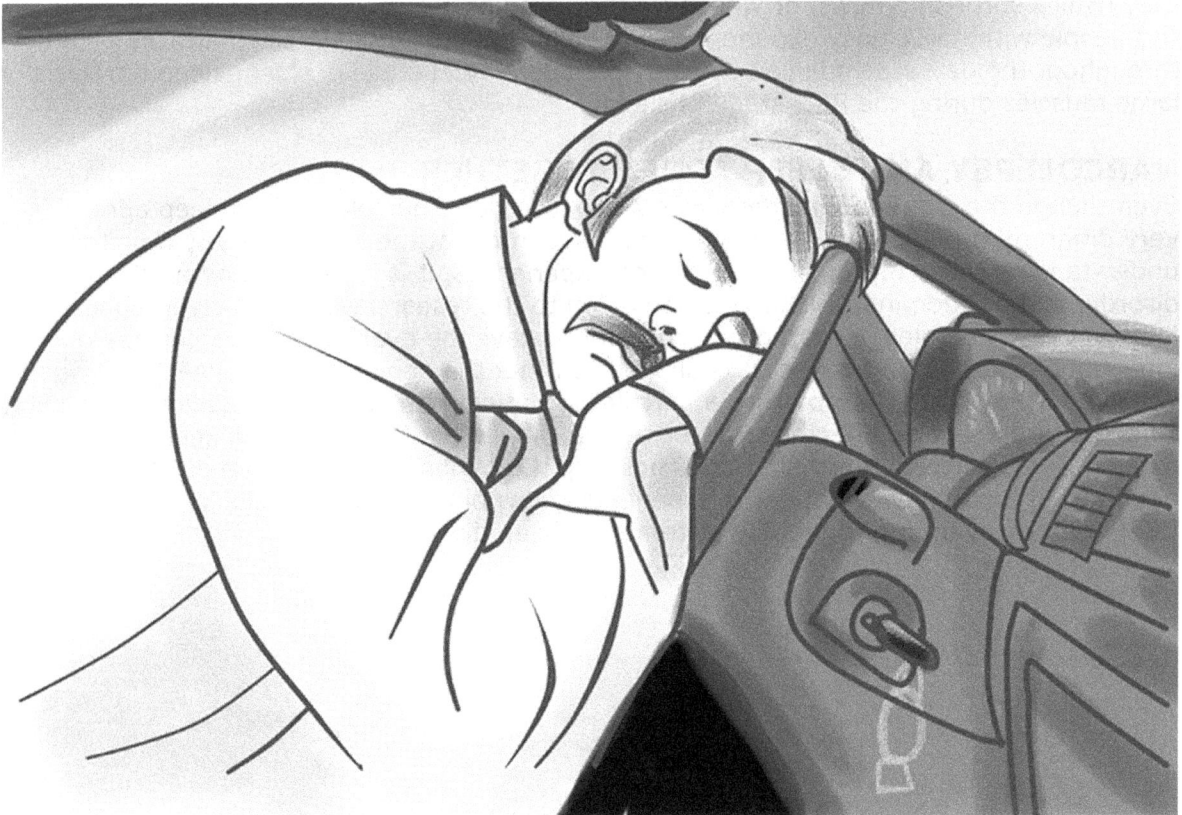

Figure 6.4 A person with narcolepsy and/or sleep apnea fell asleep on wheel while driving.

HOW IS REM STAGE OF SLEEP MONITORED?

If you are suffering from chronic insomnia, your doctor (insomnia specialist), after confirming your symptoms, may order the POLYSOMNOGRAM test in a sleep laboratory.

In a sleep disorder clinic or a sleep lab, the following tests are performed to diagnose a patient with chronic insomnia and/or sleep apnea:

Polysomnogram Test (PSG Test)

The overnight polysomnogram test is done to monitor the overall sleep of a patient during the nighttime, by monitoring sleep activities during all 5 stages of sleep including the REM sleep. This diagnostic overnight PSG also monitors a variety of body functions during the sleep, including breathing patterns, heart rhythms, heart rate, pulse rate, limb movements, snoring, percentage saturation of oxygen in the blood (SpO2) and its fluctuation throughout the sleep, and the number of sleep apnea episodes during the sleep. This test is also used to diagnose a patient with sleep apnea (mild, moderate and severe).

Multiple Sleep Latency Test (MSLT)

This test is performed usually in the morning following the overnight polysomnogram test. This test is done to diagnose if a person has been suffering from narcolepsy, and to measure the degree of daytime sleepiness. It measures how quickly you abruptly fall asleep in quiet situations during the day. It also monitors how quickly and how often you enter REM sleep. It also determines if you spent all or part of your time in REM sleep.

CPAP Titration Test

This is a two-night sleep test. On the first night the polysomnogram is done. If the patient is diagnosed with sleep apnea, the test is continued on the second night to determine the appropriate air pressure for the CPAP (Continuous Positive Airway Pressure) therapy. The compressor of the CPAP machine delivers air through a nasal mask to the patient's throat so that the airway is perfectly open throughout the night while sleeping.

HOW IS POLYSOMNOGRAM TEST DONE FOR REM SLEEP [18, 19, 20, 21]

A polysomnography is a complex procedure which serves as an essential tool for the diagnosis and understanding of sleep disorders such as sleep apnea and chronic insomnia.

It is performed by trained Registered Polysomnography Technologists (RPSGT), Registered Respiratory Therapists (RRT), EEG Technicians or by a Sleep Lab Nurse or Nurses.

Polysomnogram test involves the collection and analysis of a person's sleep physiological signals by using the appropriate electronic equipment for sleep study such as shown below:

- EEG (Electroencephalogram) to measure and record brain wave activity.
- EMG (Electromyogram) to record muscle activity such as face twitches, teeth grinding and leg movements; it also helps in determining the presence of REM stage sleep.
- EOG (Electro-Oculogram) to record REM stage sleep, eye movements; these movements are important in determining the 5 different sleep stages.
- ECG/EKG (Electrocardiogram) to record heart rate and rhythm.
- Nasal airflow sensor to record airflow.
- Snore microphone to record snoring activity.

When you arrive at the sleep lab to undergo the polysomnogram test, the technician/nurse would ask you to wait in your room until you will be called. After some time, the technician places sticky patches and sensors/electrodes on your scalp (to measure brain activity), on the outer edge of the eyelids (to capture eye movements for REM sleep), under the chin (for muscle activity), shoulders (for ECG), legs (for leg movements), face, chest, limbs and a finger. The technician would also place two elastic belts on your chest and abdomen to monitor your chest movements, and the strength and duration of the inhaled and exhaled breaths. A finger probe is used to measure blood oxygen levels and a sensor is placed in front of the nose and the mouth to measure breathing. Live video recording is used as well in some labs. After attaching all the wiring connections, you will be asked to sleep.

When you fall asleep and go into deep sleep, the thin and flexible wires connected to those sensors/electrodes would record your brain activity, eye movements, heart rate and rhythm, blood pressure, and the amount of oxygen in the blood, and electronically transmit the information to the data processor, which is connected to a computer in the nearby central processing room. A technician in the room nearby sits with a computer to make sure that all data is being recorded properly. You would not feel any discomfort during the sleep because all the wires connected to the sensors/electrodes are soft and flexible.

At the end of the test, by the next morning, the technician removes all the sensors and patches from your body and would instruct you to go home. The report will be sent to your doctor. The doctor would discuss the results with you on your next appointment.

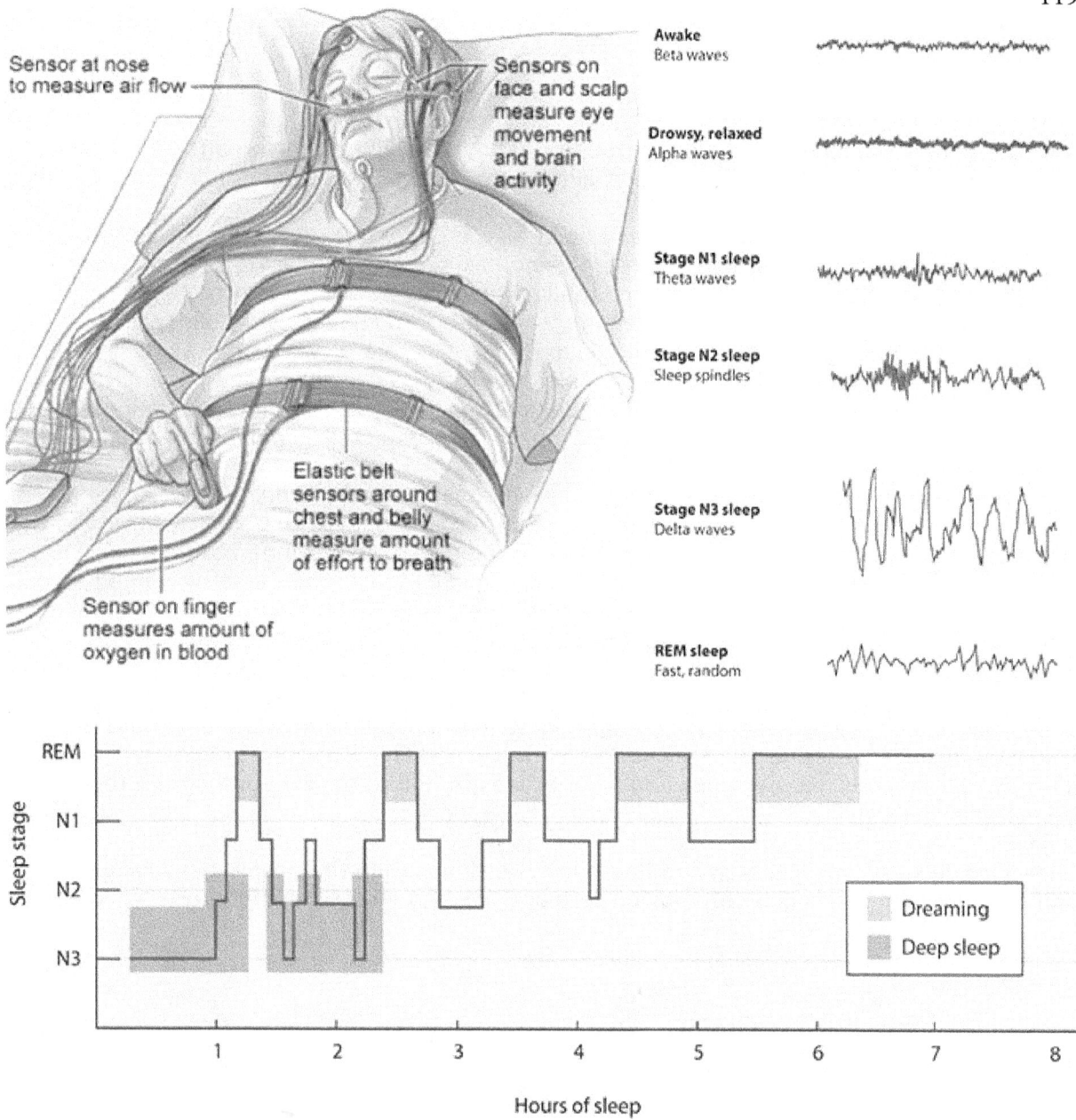

Figure 6.5 A patient is taking polysomnogram test in a sleep lab.

The chart in this page shows the polysomnogram recording (blood oxygen level versus time), breathing event versus time, and rapid eye movement (REM) versus time.
The length of the REM stage of sleep is being increased cycle after cycle in 8 hours of sleep.

IS POLYSOMNOGRAM TEST COMFORTABLE TO THE PATIENT?

♦ TOO MUCH NOISE AND BRIGHT LIGHTS IN THE SLEEP LAB COULD CAUSE INSOMNIA.

♦ The polysomnogram test should be conducted carefully in a very quiet and dark place so that the patient could fall asleep easily for at least 4 hours without being affected by any disturbance. But many hospitals do not maintain the polysomnogram lab to the comfort of patients because of lack of funding.

♦ The sleep lab is not as comfortable and quiet as the patients expect. Hospitals try to accommodate several patients in one room using dividers and by placing several beds side by side to do the polysomnogram test on multiple patients at the same time.

♦ Each patient is not completely isolated in a soundproof room and every patient could easily hear the other patients. When the technician walks to a patient, all the other patients could hear the noise of his/her footsteps. When the technician talks to one patient, all the other patients could hear the noise and because of that noisy atmosphere, some patients may not be able to fall asleep, and may not be able to complete the polysomnogram test successfully.

♦ Sometimes the air conditioner in the sleep room could be making noise. The temperature may be too hot or too cold. It may take a long time for the patient to get accustomed to the temperature. Plus not everyone is comfortable in the same room temperature.

♦ For every simple thing the patient needs, he/she needs to call the nurse by ringing a bell. The patient has no freedom to do anything, even to pass urine on his/her own. The patient may have to walk a long distance with his/her sensors attached, escorted by a nurse, to go to the bathroom.

♦ This kind of bureaucratic and irritating aspects of a hospital stay could annoy a patient and could cause insomnia. Moreover, bright lights in the hospital environment could cause insomnia in some patients.

♦ If the patient does not sleep peacefully for at least 4 hours, the polisomnogram test would be marked "INCOMPLETE".

Therefore do your own research and find out if the sleep lab in the hospital in your area is being maintained properly before going there and wasting your time and effort.

REFERENCES

1. How Dreams Work by Lee Ann Obringer, How Stuff works.
http://science.howstuffworks.com/life/inside-the-mind/human-brain/dream2.htm

2. Brain Basics: Understanding Sleep. Sleep: A Dynamic Activity, National Institute of Neurological Disorders and Stroke, National Institutes of Health, Bethesda, MD 20892, USA.
https://www.ninds.nih.gov/Disorders/Patient-Caregiver-Education/Understanding-Sleep

3. When we have REM sleep, what type of brain waves (alpha or beta) we have?
MadSci Network: Neuroscience, Posted by Benoit A. Bacon, Post-doc Fellow, Psychology Dept, University of Glasgow, Scotland, UK.
http://www.madsci.org/posts/archives/2001-03/985719909.Ns.r.html

4. Stages of Sleep, Psychology World
https://web.mst.edu/~psyworld/sleep_stages.htm
https://web.mst.edu/~psyworld/general/sleepstages/sleepstages.pdf

5. Power of Imagination Website, Written by Dr. RK.
http://www.power-of-imagination.com/

6. Brain Waves and the Deeper States of Consciousness by Tania Kotso.s
http://www.mind-your-reality.com/brain_waves.html

7. Your Hormones, Posted by Society for Endocrinology, Dec 11, 2014.
http://www.yourhormones.info/hormones/leptin.aspx

8. What is Ghrelin?, Posted by Dr. Ananya Mandal, MD, News Medical Life Sciences, Sept 17, 2014.
http://www.news-medical.net/health/What-is-Ghrelin.aspx

9. Is Lack of Sleep Making Me Fat?, by Julia Layton, Science, How Stuff Works.
http://science.howstuffworks.com/life/sleep-obesity1.htm

10. Does My Body Burn Calories While I Sleep? by Dr. Michael Breus, PhD
https://www.sharecare.com/health/metabolism-and-weight-loss/does-body-burn-calories-sleep

11. What are the Benefits of Rapid Eye Movement (REM) Sleep? by Tim Ferriss.
https://www.sharecare.com/health/sleep-disorders/what-are-benefits-rem-sleep

12. Train Your Brain to Get Thin: Prime Your Gray Cells for Weight Loss, Wellness & Exercise, by Melinda Boyd, RD and Michele Noonan, PhD, 258 pages, ISBN: 1440540152, Book Published by Adams Media of F. W. Media Inc., 2013.

13. How Sleep Works: The Sleep-Wake Cycle (Paragraph in the middle of the webpage), How to Get Better Sleep, The Beginner's Guide to Overcoming Sleep Deprivation by James Clear.
http://jamesclear.com/better-sleep

14. Sleep and Body Fat, Posted by ConfessandChillax, April 8, 2012.
https://confessandchillax.wordpress.com/2012/04/08/sleep-and-burn-fat/

122

15. Narcolepsy: A Sleep Disorder May Be Harming Your Body and Brain, Consumer Health Digest.
https://www.consumerhealthdigest.com/sleep-disorder/narcolepsy-may-harm-your-body-and-brain.html

16. Narcolepsy.
http://www.webmd.com/sleep-disorders/guide/narcolepsy#1

17. Narcolepsy And Sleep Apnea: Can You Have One When You Have The Other?, Apnea Treatment Center.
http://www.apneatreatmentcenter.com/narcolepsy-and-sleep-apnea-can-you-have-one-when-you-have-the-other/

18. How is Sleep Apnea Diagnosed by National Heart, Lung and Blood Institute.
http://www.nhlbi.nih.gov/health/health-topics/topics/slpst/during   (old link, now broken)
https://www.nhlbi.nih.gov/health/health-topics/topics/sleepapnea/diagnosis

19. Complete Polysomnography with EEG by Clinique Sommeil Santé, LaSalle – Montreal, Quebec, H8N 1Y5, Canada.
http://sommeilsante.com/services/diagnostic-lab-montreal-lasalle/

20. How A Sleep Study Works by WebMD.
http://www.webmd.com/sleep-disorders/guide/polysomnogram

21. Overnight Attended Sleep Study in the Hospital, Sleep Medicine Center, Stanford Health Care.
https://stanfordhealthcare.org/medical-clinics/sleep-medicine-center/tests/overnight--attended-sleep-study.html

CHAPTER 7: TABLE OF CONTENTS

HISTORY OF CAFFEINE

Caffeine was first discovered from the seed of a coffee cherry in 1820. [1]
Caffeine is the plant's bitter alkaloid. When extracted from the seed, it crystallizes into silky threads to form a fleecy and toxic powder. Being an addictive agent, caffeine can cause anxiety, dependency, and its overdose could lead to death.

Caffeine has been found in dozens of plants and seeds. In West Africa, kola nuts are a rich source of caffeine and have been chewed throughout history as a stimulant and strengthener. It is used today at work, in ceremony and socially. Kola can be brewed too, to make a drink called cola. Cola is one of the most popular beverages on earth. The most popular cola "Coca-Cola" was invented by Dr. John Pemberton, a pharmacist who mixed the kick of kola caffeine with the kick of coca. [1]

Coca grows in the Andean mountains of South America. Like the seeds of coffee and kola plants, coca leaves bestow the power of endurance when chewed. Coca has been used by people for thousands of years. In August 1499, Amerigo Vespucci, sailing northwest along the coast of Venezuela, encountered an island of men with the leaf tucked in their cheeks. For centuries thereafter, Europeans heard astonishing tales of the plant fueling marathons across mountains without food or rest. [1]

The word caffeine comes from the Arab word *qahwah*. The botanical name of the original species discovered in Africa whose beans are grown around the world today is Coffea Arabica. Coffee berries, the fruit of the plant, which contains the beans, are usually harvested by hand and undergo a lengthy processing procedure. Once removed from the berries, the beans are fermented, washed, dried, hulled, and peeled before they are roasted. After roasting, the Coffee beans are ground and then they are ready to perk, brew, or drip into your favorite cup of java. [2]

Caffeine is produced by more than 80 species of plants, and the reason may well be survival. As it turns out, **caffeine is a biological poison** used by plants as a pesticide. The caffeine gives seeds and leaves a bitter taste, which discourages their consumption by insects and animals. When humans consume caffeine, it does not accumulate in the bloodstream or body and is normally excreted within several hours following the consumption. In fact, only 1% of caffeine is excreted. The remaining 90% must be detoxified by the liver, and the removal of the resulting metabolites is a slow and difficult process. It can take up to 12 hours to detoxify a single cup of coffee. Evidence suggests that it can take up to 7 days to decaffeinate the blood of habitual coffee drinkers. [2]

Caffeine is a central nervous system (CNS) stimulant of the methylxanthine class. It is the world's most widely consumed, legal, unregulated and psychoactive drug. [3]

THE SOURCES OF CAFFEINE [4, 5]

Caffeine is an alkaloid occurring naturally in more than 60 plant species such as coffee beans, tea beans, cocoa beans, kola nuts, soft candy, soda, baked goods, ice cream, food supplements, energy drinks, chocolate, and many other drinks, foods and snacks. Several natural sources of caffeine include yerba maté, guarana berries, guayusa, and the yaupon holly.

CAFFEINE CONSUMPTION GUIDELINES [6, 7, 8, 9]

The maximum limit of caffeine consumption depends on the weight of the person, the sex whether male or female, and how sensitive the person is to the negative effects of caffeine. Caffeine is present not just in coffee, but also in many foods and drinks. Each person is different and so each person should do some of their own research to find out how much caffeine consumption is too much by considering all foods and drinks being consumed every day, and should not overconsume caffeine.

a. FDA (The US Food and Drug Administration) recommended in 2007 that the caffeine intake for adults should be less than 200 mg (or 1 to 2 regular cups) per day. [6]

b. A review undertaken by Health Canada scientists has considered the numerous studies dealing with caffeine and its potential health effects. It has re-confirmed that for the average adult, moderate daily caffeine intake at dose levels of 400 mg/day is not associated with any adverse effects. [7]

c. The Dietitians of Canada posted the Health Canada recommendation, saying pregnant and breastfeeding women limit their intake to no more than 300 mg per day (about two, 8oz cups of coffee or six, 8oz cups of tea). And for children aged 12 and under, a maximum daily intake should be no more than 2.5mg/kg of body weight. [8]

d. The UK Food Standards Agency has recommended that pregnant women should limit their caffeine intake to less than 200 mg of caffeine a day – the equivalent of two cups of instant coffee, or one and a half to two cups of fresh coffee. [9]

e. The American Congress of Obstetricians and Gynecologists (ACOG) concluded in 2010 that caffeine consumption is safe up to 200 mg per day in pregnant women. [9]

CAFFEINE CONSUMPTION: HOW MUCH IS TOO MUCH? [10]
ANSWER: More Than 500 mg/day Is Too Much!

American daily middle-market newspaper "USA Today" published an article revealing that: "Most people can safely take in about 400 milligrams of caffeine daily or about 4 cups of coffee, according to Robert Glatter, an emergency physician at Lenox Hill Hospital in New York City." However, this maximum limit varies from person to person, and greatly depends on the height, weight and health condition of the person.

The article also revealed that the overconsumption of caffeine **"more than 500 mg per day"** could lead to several side effects such as accelerated heart beat, muscle tremors, frequent urination, migraine headache, and stomach upset. More important side effects are insomnia, nervousness, irritability and restlessness.

IMPORTANT RECOMMENDATION: A person must research on his/her body and figure out by trial and error how much coffee is too much, and find out the optimum number of cups (1 cup, 2 cups or 3 cups) that could keep him/her alert during the day, and does not interfere with the sleep during the night. For example, the author of this book (Dr. RK) drinks 1 cup of organic coffee at 7 am, and then 1 to 2 cups of decaf before 11 am. That would keep him alert during the day and does not cause insomnia during the night. Each person must determine his/her suitable amount of coffee to be consumed.

CAFFEINE CONTENT IN FOODS AND DRINKS-I [11, 12, 13, 14]

The caffeine content in foods and drinks varies significantly and cannot be trusted. A cup of coffee here and there many not contain the same amount of caffeine. If you drink coffee in coffee-shops, Starbucks, restaurants and many other places where coffee is being sold, you should be extremely careful because the caffeine content in the coffee varies significantly from place to place and from time to time.

Scientists at the University of Florida bought a 16-oz cup of coffee of the same type from the same coffee-shop for six days straight. They analyzed each cup of coffee to determine how much caffeine it contained. They found **a wide range of caffeine levels** in the six cups of coffee. The lowest caffeine level was 259 mg and the highest was 564 mg per 16-oz cup.

Coffee's caffeine content depends on many factors. These include the type of bean that is used and how the coffee is prepared. In the same way, the size of a tea bag, number of tea-leaves and the brewing time can affect the caffeine level of a cup of tea.

Table 7.1 Caffeine content in most commonly served drinks.

S No	Beverage/Drink (1 Cup = 250 mL = 8 Oz)	Volume (mL)	Amount of Caffeine (mg)
1	Hot Chocolate	250 mL	5
2	Decaffeinated coffee	130 mL	15
3	Iced Tea/White Tea	330 mL	20
4	Green Tea	250 mL	31
5	Cola-type Soft Drink	355 mL	35
6	Caffeinated Soft Drinks	330 mL	39
7	Black Tea	250 mL	47
8	Instant Coffee	250 mL	51
9	A Chocolate Bar	100 g	65
10	Plunger Coffee	250 mL	66
11	Enery Drink	250 mL	80
12	Cappuccino	260 mL	105

CAFFEINE CONTENT IN FOODS AND DRINKS-II
WEBSITES WHERE CAFFEINE CONTENT IS LISTED

The following links, available on the Internet, would show the caffeine content in foods and drinks being sold and/or served in a variety of restaurants, coffee shops and other places. Please refer to the following websites for more information:

I. Caffeine Content in Foods & Drinks, FDA Website
https://www.fda.gov/downloads/ucm200805.pdf

II. Caffeine Chart: Caffeine Content of Foods & Beverages You Consume, Center for Science in the Public Interest
https://cspinet.org/eating-healthy/ingredients-of-concern/caffeine-chart?gclid=CjwKEAjwxurIBRDnt7P7rODiq0USJADwjt5DHk6VwIowVqqwHLNkzQIsb12KP-xiVwyewLunmJNwDxoCmSzw_wcB

III. Caffeine content in coffee, tea, soda and more by Mayo Clinic Staff
http://www.mayoclinic.org/healthy-living/nutrition-and-healthy-eating/in-depth/caffeine/art-20049372

IV. Caffeine Content in Foods & Drinks at Restaurants
http://www.nutritionmyths.com/caffeine-levels-in-drinks-and-foods/

V. Caffeine Content in Energy Drinks
http://www.webmd.com/food-recipes/news/20121025/how-much-caffeine-energy-drink#2

VI. Caffeine Content in Foods & Drinks Varies Significantly and Cannot Be Trusted, Sleep and Caffeine, Sleep Education
http://www.sleepeducation.org/news/2013/08/01/sleep-and-caffeine

VII. The 10 Most Caffeinated Diet Drinks
http://www.diet-blog.com/07/the_10_most_caffeinated_diet_drinks.php

VIII. Caffeine Content in Tim Horton's Drinks
http://www.timhortons.com/ca/en/pdf/CAFFEINE_CONTENT_-_Canada_-_August2014.pdf

Caffeine in Hot Chocolate= 15 mg (small) to 35 mg (Ex Large)

IX. Caffeine Content of Popular Drinks (National Soft Drink Association, US Food and Drug Administration, Bunker and McWilliams, Pepsi, Slim-Fast)
https://www.math.utah.edu/~yplee/fun/caffeine.html

X. Caffeine Content of Drinks by Wilstar
http://wilstar.com/caffeine.htm

XI. Caffeine in Foods and Beverages by World of Caffeine
http://worldofcaffeine.com/caffeine-in-foods-and-beverages/

129

XII. How Much Caffeine Is in Coffee, Tea, Cola, & Other Drinks?
by Lindsey Goodwin, The Spruce, Updated April 12, 2017
https://www.thespruce.com/caffeine-in-coffee-tea-cola-765276

XIII. Caffeine Content of Pre-packaged National-Brand and Private-Label
Carbonated Beverages, Wiley Online Library
http://onlinelibrary.wiley.com/doi/10.1111/j.1750-3841.2007.00414.x/abstract

XIV. Hot Chocolate Contains Only a Little Caffeine
http://www.livestrong.com/article/264573-caffeine-in-hot-chocolate-vs-coffee/

XV. Does Hot Chocolate Contains Caffeine?
Caffeine Content of Some Popular Drinks (List)
http://www.newhealthadvisor.com/Does-Hot-Chocolate-Have-Caffeine.html

XVI. Caffeine Content in Energy Drinks by Caffeine Informer
http://www.caffeineinformer.com/the-caffeine-database

XVII. Caffeine Amounts in Soda: Every Kind of Cola You Can Think Of by
Caffeine Informer
https://www.caffeineinformer.com/caffeine-amounts-in-soda-every-kind-of-cola-you-can-think-of

XVIII. Caffeine Levels in Slurpee by Caffeine Informer;
Some Slurpee Flavors Have Caffeine in Them
A Slurpee is a Popular Frozen Drink Available at 7-Eleven Convenience Stores.
https://www.caffeineinformer.com/caffeine-content/slurpee-frozen-drinks

XIX. How Much Caffeine Is in Decaf Coffee?
https://www.healthline.com/nutrition/caffeine-in-decaf#what-it-is

LIMITED CAFFEINE CONSUMPTION HAS POSITIVE EFFECTS [15, 27]

Overconsumption of caffeine over time leads to addiction, sleep disorder, fatigue and pain. But scientists believe that limited caffeine consumption has positive effects.

Recent studies (some 19,000) suggested that coffee and caffeine may actually offer some significant medical benefits. Those studies have uncovered a range of positive effects that caffeine seems to have on the human body: [27]

♦ Regular coffee drinkers were 80 percent less likely to develop Parkinson's disease.
♦ Two cups a day reduced the subjects' risk for colon cancer by 20 percent.
♦ Two cups a day caused an 80 percent drop in the odds of developing cirrhosis.
♦ Two cups a day cut the risk of developing gallstones in half.
♦ Caffeine is beneficial in treating asthma, stopping headaches, boosting mood and even preventing cavities
♦ Researchers are developing drugs for Parkinson's disease containing caffeine and caffeine-derivatives.
♦ A study by the Byrd Alzheimer's Institute in Tampa, Fla., showed that lab mice injected with caffeine were protected against developing Alzheimer's disease. The injections even helped reduce symptoms in those that had the disease. The findings lead doctors to believe that up to five cups of coffee a day could have the same positive effect on humans.
♦ A 2007 study at Rutgers University suggested that regular exercise combined with daily doses of caffeine could increase the destruction of precancerous skin cells in mice. Once again, the findings have not yet been tested on humans, but the indication is that it will have similar effects.

While doctors still recommend moderate caffeine consumption, no research findings yet outlined with confidence the long-term positive or negative effects of caffeine consumption.

WebMD posted an article on the Internet suggesting that moderate consumption of caffeine is not addictive, does not cause insomnia, does not increase the risk of osteoporosis, heart disease and cancer, is not harmful for women trying to get pregnant, does not have a dehydrating effect, does not harm children, etc. [15]

For detailed information of the aforementioned recommendations, click on the following links and read through:

I.   Caffeine Myth No. 1: Caffeine Is Addictive
II.   Caffeine Myth No. 2: Caffeine Is Likely to Cause Insomnia
III.   Caffeine Myth No. 3: Caffeine Increases the Risk of Osteoporosis, Heart Disease, and Cancer
IV.   Caffeine Myth No. 4: Caffeine Is Harmful for Women Trying to Get Pregnant
V.   Caffeine Myth No. 5: Caffeine Has a Dehydrating Effect
VI.   Caffeine Myth No. 6: Caffeine Harms Children, Who, Today, Consume Even More Than Adults
VII.   Caffeine Myth No. 7: Caffeine Can Help You Sober Up
VIII. Caffeine Myth No. 8: Caffeine Has No Health Benefits

7 Unbelievable Facts About Caffeine [16]

#1. CAFFEINE INCREASES ALERTNESS: After a morning cup of coffee, the 'zombie' awakens and can pump out morning emails and tasks and become a productive human once again. Adenosine, a neurotransmitter in the body, can play a role in making a human sleepy and caffeine will 'block' this type of activity within the nervous system.

#2. CAFFEINE IMPROVES METABOLISM: Caffeine stimulates the central nervous system of the body, sending messages that tell fat cells to break down stored fat as well as increasing the resting metabolic rate (RMR) by up to 11%. The positive effects on metabolism that caffeine creates are best felt by people who are not obese. This theory was supported by a study by the American Journal of Physiology that found fat-burning rates could increase as much as 29% in lean or athletic individuals and 10% in obese people.

#3. CAFFEINE HELPS YOU CHEAT DEATH: Some studies showed that a daily cup of coffee can lower the risk of premature death by up to 15%. One such study, from the American Heart Association medical journal, concluded that higher intake of coffee, whether caffeinated or decaffeinated, was associated with a lower risk of total mortality.

#4. CAFFEINE CAN HINDER INTROVERTS AND HELP PERFORM EXTROVERTS: Caffeine can affect a person differently due to some factors such as age, weight, height, and health of the individual but surprisingly, personality types will also determine the effects that caffeine has on the human body. People with extrovert personality will be more likely to complete the assigned tasks easier under the influence of caffeine.

#5. CAFFEINE CAN BOOST YOUR MEMORY: John Hopkins University of Baltimore, Maryland, conducted a study comparing the recollections between two groups of people. They were asked to memorize some images and the images were slightly altered later. Both groups were brought back after 24 hours and were questioned if the images were altered or not. The group that consumed caffeine noticed the changes in images but the second group that did not consume caffeine failed to recognize the changes in the images, indicating the fact that the caffeine consumption boosts the memory.

#6. CAFFEINE PROMOTES BOWEL MOVEMENTS: Cafeeine has the relaxing ability of colonic muscles and makes the bowel movement easier. Peristalsis is the name of the process when the intestinal muscles contract and relax, allowing bowel movements, and the effect of coffee on this process is similar to that of eating a meal. Drinking coffee can also have a positive impact on those with constipation, loosening stools and making sure the body discharges the waste on a regular basis.

#7. CAFFEINE CAN KEEP YOU IN GOOD MOOD: A recent ten-year study published in the Archives of Internal Medicine (now known as JAMA) shows that women who consume 2 or 3 cups of caffeinated coffee per day were 15% less likely to develop depression than those who consumed less than 1 cup per day.

POSITIVE EFFECTS OF CAFFEINE [17, 18]

Research showed that limited caffeine consumption has positive effects in treating the following health problems: [17]

1. Parkinson's disease
2. Alzheimer's disease
3. Type-2 diabetes
4. Gallstones
5. Cancer
6. Asthma
7. Heart rhythm
8. Stroke
9. Liver disease
10. Improves the effectiveness of certain types of painkillers.

Limited Caffeine Consumption Has the Following Beneficial Effects [18]

1. It improves concentration, alertness, reasoning and vigilance
2. Helps you overcome the post-lunch dip
3. Can help the body to cope with physical exertion
4. Increases the body's level of adrenaline – the 'fight or flight' hormone to cope with dangerous or exacting situations
5. Caffeine doesn't build up in the body, as it is excreted in urine

NEGATIVE EFFECTS OF CAFFEINE [17]

Research also showed that overconsumption of caffeine has the following negative effects on the well-being of a person:

♦ Negatively affects on sleep-wake cycle
♦ Some people reported that it may cause auditory hallucinations
♦ Hampers absorption of minerals such as iron, zinc, magnesium and some vitamins
♦ Could raise blood pressure or hypertension
♦ The diuretic effect (increased urination) could lead to dehydration and loss of vitamin-B, vitamin-C, iron, calcium & zinc.
♦ It can stain your teeth
♦ The acid content of caffeine could aggravate heartburn

Overconsumption of Caffeine Could Also Cause the Following Harmful Effects [18]

♦ Can cause sleeplessness, nerviness and restlessness
♦ Being diuretic, it could make your body increase output of water
♦ Being a vasoconstrictor, it could cause your blood vessels in the body to temporarily narrow, thereby raising blood pressure
♦ Could cause headaches
♦ It has been reported by some people that it brings on panic attacks and palpitations
♦ It could be addictive if you rely on it everyday
♦ It could impede the control of fine motor movements and stimulation of urination (also called diuretic effect).

MORE NEGATIVE EFFECTS OF CAFFEINE [19]

Researchers Narula and others reported the following findings with regard to negative effects of excessive use of caffeine on human health:

1. Osteoporosis: Excessive use of caffeine reduces calcium density in bones, thus increasing the risk of diseases like osteoporosis. It was reported that 6 ounces of coffee or caffeine rich beverages can reduce up to 5mg of calcium from bones.

2. Insomnia: As caffeine imitates the structure and shape of adenosine, it increases the working capacity of a person. However, excessive use of caffeine can result in loss of sleep or insomnia, which adversely affects on human health.

3. Fertility: The study also reported that women who consume large quantities of caffeine on a daily basis are more prone to miscarriages and fertility issues. The neurochemical substance disturbs menstrual cycles in women and has serious impacts on the production of eggs.

Caffeine Overdose Symptoms [20, 21, 22, 23, 24]

Overconsumption of caffeine for prolonged periods of time from "coffee, tea, other beverages or drinks, and from many foods and snacks" disrupts sleep-wake cycle and causes insomnia, anxiety, increased muscle tension, chronic pain, fatigue and the people feel the some or more of the symptoms shown below:

Table 7.2 Caffeine overdose symptoms.

Caffeine Overdose Symptoms	
Central Part of the Body (Within the Brain) ♦ Irritability ♦ Anxiety ♦ Restlessness ♦ Confusion ♦ Delirium ♦ Headache ♦ Chronic Insonia	**Heart of the Body** ♦ Rapid Heartbeat ♦ Irregular rhythm **Respiratory Symptoms** ♦ Rapid Breathing **Urinary Symptoms** ♦ Frequent urination
Gastric Symptoms (Stomach) ♦ Abdominal Pain ♦ Nausea ♦ Vomiting Possibly with Blood	**Musclur Parts of the Body** ♦ Seizures ♦ Trembling ♦ Twitching ♦ Overextension
Systemic Symptoms ♦ Dehydration ♦ Fever	**Visual Symptoms on Eyes** ♦ Seeing Flashes
Skin Surface Symptoms ♦ Increased sensitivity ♦ Pain when touching	**Hearing Symptoms in Ears** ♦ Tinnitus (Ringing or Buzzing in the ears)

OVERCONSUMPTION OF CAFFEINE IS DANGEROUS [25, 26]

DEATH REPORTS

Caffeine, if overconsumed, can cause death. By drinking coffee, coffee pills, caffeine powder, and energy drinks loaded with caffeine, there were many deaths reported in USA and UK. There could be many more deaths unreported and undocumented around the world. With underlying medical condition, people are more susceptible to caffeine overdose. **Caffeine Informer Staff** posted the following reported deaths due to caffeine overdose:

I. CAFFEINE PILLS [25]

Caffeine pills are dangerous as they deliver a huge dose of caffeine that can be taken multiple times in a short period of time.

1. 19-year-old James Stone was found dead of caffeine toxicity after consuming a dose of two dozen No-Doz-Caffeine-Tablets, which is an equivalent dosage of 4800 mg of caffeine.

2. 26-year-old, Gemma Ann Jones from UK, was found dead after she consumed 50-100 caffeine-laden pills called EPH25. It appears that this caffeine death was a suicide.

3. Another woman from UK, Katie Goard, also recently overdosed by taking diet pills, called Fat Metaboliser. An autopsy revealed that Katie consumed caffeine that could be an equivalent to more than 50 cups of coffee.

4. 24-year-old Cara Reynolds from UK recently overdosed on raspberry ketone pills. Each pill contained 160 mg of caffeine. This was an intentional overdose due to her mental state after breaking up with her boyfriend.

II. CAFFEINE POWDER [25]

5. An Ohio teenager, Logan Stiner, was found dead after ingesting a large dose of pure caffeine powder. The coroner said that the young man's blood had a caffeine concentration of 70 micrograms per milliliter of blood. (The normal level of caffeine is 1-15 micrograms per milliliter of blood).

III. ENERGY DRINKS [25]

6. A 28-year-old patient, with a pre-medical condition, suffered a fatal cardiac arrest after consuming an unnamed caffeinated energy drink.

7. A Nigerian man died after drinking 8 cans of Bullet Energy Drink.

8. A Japanese man died of caffeine overdose after drinking too many energy drinks along with possible intake of some caffeine pills.

9. In 2017, a 16-year-old high school student, Davis Allen Cripe died after consuming too much caffeine from several caffeine-containing drinks such as McDonald's latte, Mountain Dew drink and an unnamed energy drink. [26]

10. The FDA has been investigating some 13 deaths that could have occurred from consuming the over-the counter 5-Hour-Energy-Shot.

IV. MONSTER DRINK [25]

11. In 2011, a 14-year-old girl, after consuming two 24-ounce cans of Monster, died.

12. In 2013, a mother filed a lawsuit against Monster for the death of her 19-year-old son. He consumed 3 Monsters in 24 hours, and then died.

13. In 2015, a 19-year-old teenager reportedly drank 3 1/2 twenty-four fluid ounce Monsters and then played basketball. He collapsed while playing and died at the hospital. His father is now suing Monster (in January 2017).

CAFFEINE IS ADDICTIVE: HERE IS WHY!

[27, 28, 29, 30, 31, 32, 33, 34, 35, 36, 37]

Adenosine is a chemical substance in the brain that binds to specific receptors. Its purpose is to make a person feel tired and sleepy by the end of the day. Caffeine on the other hand has the stimulating effect on the brain, boosts a person's mood and makes a person alert whenever a person consumes it.

Caffeine, by having similar shape and chemical structure to adenosine molecules, can also bind the same adenosine receptors in the brain whenever a person consumes caffeine-containing food or drink. When a person consumes coffee in the morning, the caffeine molecules enter the bloodstream, compete and occupy the adenosine receptors in the brain by pushing the adenosine molecules away from the their receptors. Then the person remain alert upon consuming coffee.

As the coffeine molecules continually compete and block adenosine molecules, overtime, the brain generates more adenosine receptors in order to facilitate the adenosine molecules. To keep the adenosine molecules from occupying the new adenosine receptors, the brain demands more and more coffee, and relies on more caffeine molecules to plug up the new receptors. Therefore the person becomes addictive to coffee to remain alert.

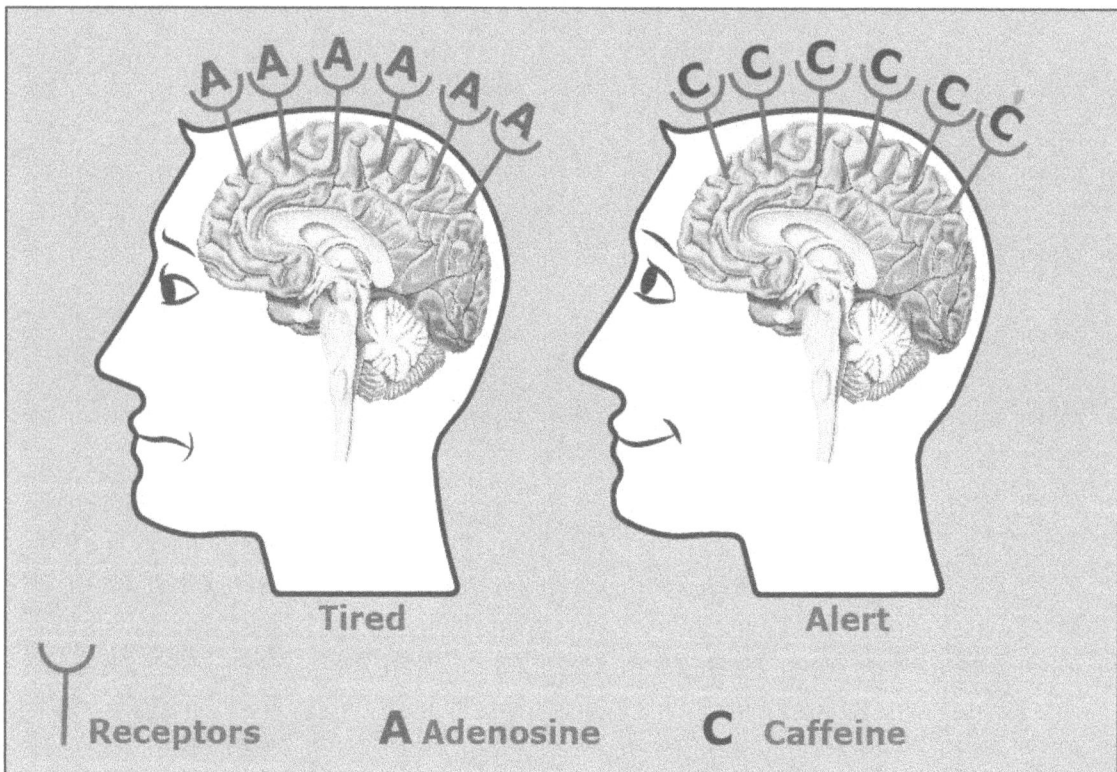

Figure 7.1 How caffeine molecules occupy adenosine receptors on the brain.

YouTube Video Posted By Mitchell Moffit and Gregory Brown Who Demystify How Caffeine Is Addictive [27]

Watch the Following YouTube Video Titled "Your Brain On Coffee."
https://www.youtube.com/watch?v=4YOwEqGykDM

Mitchell Moffit and Gregory Brown demystified the inner workings of caffeine in their latest ASAP Science video. Watch the animation on the video to understand how caffeine molecules replace adenosine molecules in the receptors of your brain to make you alert.

THE STIMULATING EFFECT OF COFFEE ON YOUR BRAIN: Naturally when you work throughout the day, a chemical called adenosine is accumulated, binds and occupy the adenosine-receptors on your brain, and slows down brain activity, making you feel fatigued. The more adenosine is accumulated, the more tired and sleepy your brain feels. Conversely, as the night progresses and as you rest and sleep, the concentration of adenosine declines, gradually promoting wakefulness by the morning. But it turns out that the caffeine in the coffee you drink is incredibly very similar to adenosine in chemical structure. When you drink coffee, the caffeine gets into the blood stream, and then into your brain, and hijacks and competes with the adenosine molecules, occupy adenosine-receptors by pushing them out of their receptors. But because adenosine-receptors are occupied by caffeine molecules, your brain does not feel sleepy, but feels stimulated by the caffeine. As you are on coffee for long time, your brain generates more adenosine-receptors, allowing adenosine to get back into the receptors. In order to keep the adenosine molecules away from those new receptors and to keep you alert, your brain demands more coffee to drink, and as a result you become addicted to coffee. Also, if you missed your daily dose of coffee you may feel more tired than you would otherwise because of the increased amount of adenosine receptors sending the 'sleepy signals' to your brain. [28, 29]

Caffeine also stimulates the production of adrenaline by the pituitary gland. Adrenaline increases heart rate, gets the blood pumping, opens airways, and even prevents reabsorption of dopamine into the brain, making you feel more happy. It is this level of stimulation that makes coffee so addictive. [30]

This exact same concept was reviewed and posted by TheJournal.ie of Ireland [28], Lauren F Friedman [29] and Tobeagenius. [30]

Review Posted By Joseph Stromberg [31]

Caffeine is a central nervous system (CNS) stimulant of the methylxanthine class. It is the world's most widely consumed psychoactive drug, which is legal to consume in nearly all parts of the world. [3] Like many drugs such as heroin, cannabis/marijuana, cocaine, tobacco or even alcohol, caffeine is chemically addictive. Given below is the explanation.

When we consume caffeine-containing food, drink or coffee, caffeine is absorbed through the small intestine and dissolved into the bloodstream. Caffeine is both water-soluble (which means it can easily dissolve in a water-based solution such as blood), and fat-soluble, which means it penetrates into the body's cell membranes, and it also enters the blood-brain barrier, a filtering mechanism of the capillaries that carry blood to the brain and spinal cord tissue, blocking the passage of certain substances before entering the brain. The amount of caffeine in the bloodstream peaks 15 to 45 minutes after ingestion (each person of course is different).

In human brain, adenosine molecules are produced by our daily activities and they stay attached to adenosine-receptors. Adenosine protects us by slowing nerve cell activity. Adenosine works to naturally trigger tiredness so that we become sleepy and rest. There are four types of adenosine receptors (A1, A2a, A2b, A3). The receptors A1 and A2a regulate the release of the neurotransmitters such as dopamine and glutamate.

However the caffeine molecule and adenosine molecule possess a similar chemical structure as shown below:

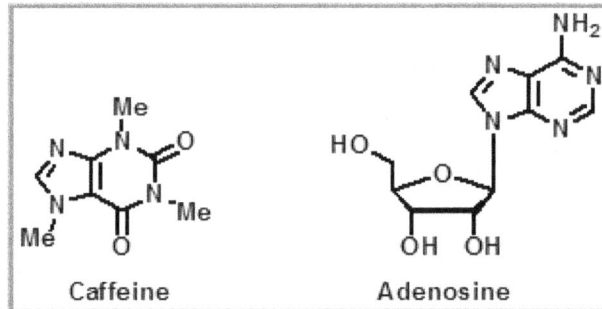

Figure 7.2 The chemical structure of caffeine and adenosine.

Caffeine molecules, as they look like adenosine molecules, easily bind to the adenosine-receptors, thereby blocking the adenosine molecules to enter the receptors. That means caffeine molecules occupy the adenosine-receptors and replace the adenosine whenever we drink coffee and as soon as the caffeine enters the brain. But adenosine and caffeine exhibit opposite effects. Caffeine therefore not only blocks adenosine's ability to slow nerve activity, but increases the nerve activity, leaving a person stimulated, more alert, energetic for a few hours, which the caffeine drinkers crave and which makes them addicted. Caffeine, if consumed excessively, could cause jitters (feeling of extreme nervousness, tension and anxiety).

CAFFEINE ALSO STIMULATES THE PRODUCTION OF ADRENALINE AND DOPAMINE:
By blocking adenosine molecules in the brain, caffeine also promotes the brain's production of two natural stimulants dopamine and glutamine, which help boost our mood and alertness, and even reduce the risk of depression for some people. When adenosine-receptors are blocked by caffeine molecules, all the surplus adenosine floating around in the brain instructs the adrenal glands, which are located on the top of the kidneys, to secrete and flood another fight-or-flight hormone (fight-or-flight means the instinctive physiological response to a threatening situation, which readies one either to resist forcibly or to run away), a powerful stimulant and neurotransmitter called adrenaline (epinephrine) all over the body. [33]

Adrenaline has a number of effects on your body:
♦ Your pupils dilate so you will have an illusion of heightened alertness.
♦ The airway opens up (this is why people suffering from severe asthma attacks are sometimes injected with epinephrine).
♦ Your heart beats faster and heart rate increases.
♦ Blood vessels on the surface constrict to slow down the blood flow from cuts and increase blood flow to muscles instead.
♦ Blood pressure rises.
♦ Blood flow to the stomach slows down.
♦ The liver releases sugar into the bloodstream for giving you extra energy.
♦ Muscles tighten up, and get ready for action.

Dopamine (and also glutamine) is another neurotransmitter that activates pleasure centers in certain parts of the brain. The most addictive so-called street-drugs heroin and cocaine manipulate and promote dopamine levels, inducing "ecstasy" into the person's brain. Caffeine increases dopamine levels, stimulates the brain and induces alertness in the same manner. Its effect is much weaker than heroin's, but the mechanism is the same. Researchers believe that it is the dopamine connection that makes a person addicted to caffeine, very similar to the drugs heroine and cocaine. [33] It is therefore that caffeine is not believed to be a stimulant itself, but it is stimulant-enabler.

But caffeine can cause a vicious cycle of problems in the long term. For example, once caffeine-induced adrenaline wears off, you face low-energy levels, fatigue and even depression. Another cup of coffee or energy drink can get the adrenaline flowing again, but having your body in a state of emergency, jumpy and irritable all day long, is not very healthy. [11] Adrenaline has the ability to make us more irritable and emotionally unstable.

The long-term effect of caffeine is "sleep deprivation." Caffeine if consumed excessively effects sleep-wake cycle and causes chronic insomnia. Caffeine has half-life of 6 hours. That means if you consume a large cup of coffee containing 200 mg of caffeine at around 3 pm, half of that caffeine (100 mg) would be ingested and eliminated from your body in 6 hours, and the remaining half (another 100 mg) would stay in your body for 12 hours (till 3 am) effecting your sleep. You will end up tossing and turning instead of sleeping, and you may miss the benefits of deep sleep and REM sleep because of the presence of caffeine in your system. The next morning you wake up tired and dissatisfied with your sleep, once again desperately wanting to drink coffee to be more alert. The following night would be even worse and you will continue suffering from sleep deprivation. This cycle would continue exactly like a chain reaction, and you become addicted to caffeine.

If you quit coffee, the **withdrawal symptoms** would be devastating. You would feel mentally foggy, lack alertness, be in a depressed mood and have difficulty concentrating. Your muscles could be fatigued and would suffer from increased muscle tension and even serious pain, and you would be more irritable than usual. You could be drowsy and will not feel like doing anything for around 48 hours. So, you will be tempted to drink coffee again unless you are a master of high willpower and high self-discipline.

If you really know how to practice and implement high willpower and high self-discipline, you would not have been in this drastic situation with the overconsumption of caffeine. Had you been drinking strictly one or two cups of coffee before noon (not in the afternoon), and had you been extremely careful by not consuming any other caffeine from any other foods and drinks, you would not have faced the problem with caffeine addiction.

Review Posted By Ari Whitten [32]

To understand the action of caffeine on brain, you first have to know what exactly the adenosine is. Adenosine is an inhibitory neurotransmitter in the Central Nervous System (CNS) that makes you tired and sleepy. Adenosine is built up from the day's biochemical activities, gets into the adenosine receptors, and as the night begins, it plays a role in letting you know when it is time to stop working and prepare to sleep. The more adenosine is accumulated in your body, the more you feel sleepy, fatigued, etc.

Caffeine works against adenosine by inhibiting the action of adenosine, which means the stimulating properties of caffeine make you feel alert and energized to work (exactly opposite to becoming sleepy). When you consume coffee or caffeine-containing substances, you now have caffeine which is also floating around inside the brain. Caffeine is in the same, or a very similar, shape as the adenosine molecule and it also fits into the adenosine receptors. When you drink coffee, caffeine will go in and hijack the adenosine receptors. This blocks the adenosine from getting into the receptors and in order to make you tried, which is why you feel energized when you drink coffee.

When you introduce caffeine into the system, it basically blocks adenosine from getting in and activating this receptor. When the adenosine receptors plugged up by caffeine, the brain then acts like there is a lot less adenosine in the system. It does not detect that adenosine is there. The adenosine is still floating around but it can not get to the receptors in the brain because of the caffeine that is blocking it.

By blocking the fatiguing effect of adenosine, the caffeine of the coffee you drink creates an energizing stimulant effect. In other words, you are blocking something which would make you tired, so by doing that, it creates a stimulant effect. That is why caffeine works as a stimulant.

Basically, more caffeine means that less adenosine is reaching the brain which makes you feel more awake and energized. When caffeine is present your brain detects less adenosine and you get more energy, more alertness, better performance, etc.

Caffeine stimulates neuron activity in the brain. Each time you drink a cup of coffee, neurons send messages to your pituitary gland which in turn alerts your adrenals to pump out adrenaline and cortisol.

To learn more about **HOW AND WHY CAFFEINE IS ADDICTIVE**, go to the websites of references 27, 28, 29, 30, 31, 32, 33, 34, 35, 36, 37 and read the contents.

CAFFEINE CAUSES SLEEP DISTURBANCES & INSOMNIA

JOURNAL PUBLICATIONS DISCUSSED

I. The Following Information Was Published in the Journal of Clinical Sleep, After Conducting the Clinical Research: [38]

This study demonstrated that caffeine consumption even 6 hours before bedtime can have important disruptive effects on both objective and subjective measure of sleep. These findings provide empirical support for sleep hygiene recommendations to refrain from substantial caffeine use for a minimum of 6 hours prior to bedtime.

Results demonstrated a moderate dose of caffeine at bedtime, 3 hours prior to bedtime, or 6 hours prior to bedtime each have significant effects on sleep disturbance relative to placebo. The magnitude of reduction in total sleep time suggests that caffeine taken 6 hours before bedtime has important disruptive effects on sleep and provides empirical support for sleep hygiene recommendations to refrain from substantial caffeine use for a minimum of 6 hours prior to bedtime.

The results of this study suggests that 400 mg of caffeine taken 0, 3, or even 6 hours prior to bedtime significantly disrupts sleep. Even after 6 hours of consumption, caffeine reduced sleep by more than 1 hour. This degree of sleep loss, if experienced over multiple nights, may have detrimental effects on daytime body function.

II. Effect of Caffeine on Sleep EEG Study in Late Middle Age People, Published by Sleep Laboratory, University of Edinburgh, Scotland [39]

Abstract

1. The effect of caffeine alkaloid base (300 mg) on a whole night's sleep was investigated by electrophysiological techniques in six late middle age subjects (mean age 56 years), comparison being made with decaffeinated coffee and with no drink prior to sleep, using each condition five times in a balanced order on non-consecutive nights.
2. After caffeine the mean total sleep time decreased on an average by 2 hours, the mean sleep latency increased to 66 minutes. The number of awakenings increased and the mean total intervening wakefulness was more than double, after caffeine consumption.
3. In the first 3 hours of sleep, a decreased amount of stage 3 + 4 was observed, accompanied by an increased amount of stage 2 and of intervening wakefulness, without a significant change in the amount of rapid eye movement sleep.
4. The change in sleep pattern observed suggests an increased capability for arousal and decreased ability to develop or sustain deeper stages of non-rapid eye movement sleep after caffeine.

Complete Article

https://www.ncbi.nlm.nih.gov/pmc/articles/PMC1402564/pdf/brjclinpharm00282-0023.pdf

III. Study Finds: Afternoon Coffee Disrupts Sleep, Posted by NHS Choices of the Government UK, 2013 [40]

Some shop-bought coffees contain up to 500mg of caffeine.
"Drinking even one cup of strong coffee in the afternoon can knock an hour off your sleep," Mail Online reports. The headline is based on a small study that tested the effects of a 400mg caffeine pill taken either at bedtime, or three or six hours before.

Researchers found that the caffeine dose (similar to that of a large shop-bought coffee) appeared to disrupt sleep even when taken six hours before bedtime. The caffeine reduced the total amount of time volunteers slept by about an hour. This effect was seen regardless of when the caffeine pill was taken.

It is important to bear in mind that the study only included a very small number of people, all of whom were generally healthy and did not have problems with sleep. The findings need to be confirmed in larger studies with more mixed groups of people of different ages to be sure of exactly how long the effects of caffeine last. Overall, the study suggests that caffeine may have an effect up to six hours before going to bed. For people concerned about having a good night's sleep, it is probably best to avoid caffeine close to when you go to bed.

Conclusion

This study suggested that caffeine intake may affect sleep even if taken six hours before bedtime. The main strengths of the study were the use of a randomized and blinded design, and the use of both self-reported and objective measures of sleep.

However, there are also limitations to the study:
- The study was very small and included a very select group of participants. It analyzed data from only 12 healthy young to middle-aged adults who took each of the timed test doses of caffeine on one night only. Larger studies in more mixed populations would be needed to confirm the findings and see if they apply to other groups.
- Not all of the self-reported and objective measurements of sleep completely agreed. For example, caffeine taken six hours before sleep only had a statistically significant effect on the objective measure of total sleep time, but not self-reported sleep time. The researchers suggest that this difference may be as a result of people having broken sleep, which they notice less than if they take longer to fall asleep, for example. Larger studies where people undergo more extensive measurements in a sleep lab may help confirm the effects.
- The average caffeine consumption of participants was about 100mg per day – about one home-brewed 8 fl oz cup of coffee. Other studies would be needed to see if the effect of the caffeine dose used in the study (400mg) differed in people who were used to consuming more or less caffeine.

Despite these limitations, if you are having problems sleeping, it makes sense to try limiting your consumption of stimulants, such as foods and drinks that contain caffeine, especially in the evening, to see if this helps.

IV. Caffeine-Induced Sleep Disorder (from Wikipedia) [41]

Caffeine increases episodes of wakefulness, and high doses in the late evening can increase sleep onset latency. In elderly people, there is an association between use of medication containing caffeine and difficulty in falling asleep.

Overconsumption: Excessive ingestion of caffeine can lead to a state of intoxication. This period of intoxication is characterized by restlessness, agitation, excitement, rambling thoughts or speech, and even insomnia. Even doses of caffeine relating to just one cup of coffee can increase sleep latency and decrease the quality of sleep especially in non-REM deep sleep. A dose of caffeine taken in the morning can have these effects the following night, so one of the main practices of sleep hygiene is to cease the consumption of caffeine.

V. Cortisol Levels – How Caffeine Intake Affects Stress Hormones, Posted by Diane Mohlman, Diet & Nutrition [42]

Adrenaline, noradrenaline and cortisol are called stress hormones. Stress increases the cortisol level. Some of the symptoms of elevated cortisol are fatigue, excess body fat and the inability to lose body fat (regardless of diet and exercise). These symptoms don't occur overnight and you may have had years of accumulated stress and it finally caught up with you. Cortisol raises the level of glucose. Excess glucose stores body fat and so now you are fatigued, carrying around excess belly fat, and can not seem to lose weight no matter what you try and how long you run on a treadmill. This is not a good position to be in!

Caffeine is a stimulant and induces stress, which in turn raises cortisol levels. A rise in cortisol will create a reaction in your body releasing amino acids from muscles, glucose from your liver, fatty acids into your blood stream and tons of energy for your survival.

The effect of caffeine, which causes stress and increases cortisol levels could develop gastrointestinal problems. When caffeine elevates cortisol levels, the energy would be taken away from our gastrointestinal tract, thereby lowering the amount of enzymes we need to digest the food we consume. The same action would also lower the minerals and nutrients in our body. Low minerals along with high acid could lead to osteoporosis.

Cortisol has an adverse effect on serotonin and dopamine production. The precursor to melatonin is serotonin, a neurotransmitter that itself is derived from the amino acid tryptophan. Within the pineal gland, serotonin is acetylated and then methylated to yield melatonin. Therefore when the cortisol level is raised due to high stress levels, the melatonin production is depleted in the night, causing sleep disturbances and even the insomnia.

Also the lack of sleep causes a very sharp increase in cortisol levels. This would draw you to the addiction of caffeine consumption for temporary energy. High levels of cortisol depletes the adrenal glands and predisposes you to chronic fatigue. High caffeine consumption elevates stress, which further elevates the cortisol levels, and thus you become a caffeine-addict. Cortisol levels should be low during the nighttime. High cortisol levels during the nighttime cause sleep disturbances, and the whole cycle would repeat exactly like a chain reaction.

VI. If You Want to Sleep Better? First, Reduce Your Cortisol Levels Then Follow These Six Key Tips, Posted by Body-Ecology [43]

Known or unknown stress or fear elevates cortisol levels. Elevated cortisol levels cause sleep disturbances and even insomnia. Cortisol is called the stress hormone, and some times it is even the called death hormone. Whenever your body goes into the fight-or-flight-response mode, cortisol is made in your adrenal glands, situated on the top of your kidneys.

For many of us, our thoughts are on overdrive and our minds are constantly filled with negative chatter. Anxiety, worry and concern cause fear and that fear can consume us and promote us to live with constant stress. When you live a life full of chronic fear, your adrenal glands, your kidneys and your bladder are weakened. As they become weakened, you will find yourself becoming even more fearful, start living with stress, and generate lots of stress hormone "cortisol". It's a vicious cycle and becomes a chain reaction and ruins your health unless you take control of your body and mind and break the cycle.

High cortisol (stress hormone) has the following negative effects on your health:
- Cortisol creates chronic to severe inflammation that eventually causes premature aging and leads to an earlier death.
- Cortisol suppresses the important youth hormones DHEA, testosterone & estrogen.
- Cortisol causes blood sugar levels to elevate. This then leads to an acidic blood condition. Acidic blood leads to diabetes, heart disease and also cancer.
- Lowered immunity
- Poor short-term memory
- Constipation
- Weight gain, especially in the abdominal region and the waist
- Loss of muscle tone
- Osteoporosis (a medical condition in which the bones become brittle and fragile from loss of tissue, typically as a result of hormonal changes, or deficiency of calcium or vitamin D)

Six Tips to Manage Fear and Elevated Cortisol:

A few simple lifestyle changes, together with nutritional nourishment for your adrenals and some special herbs called adaptogens will help you obtain a much deeper level of sleep at night.

1. Make an Effort to Grow Emotionally Happier. Practice EFT (Emotional Freedom Technique).
2. Make An Effort to Grow Spiritually. Become spiritual and learn to meditate.
3. Make Some Simple Changes in the Way You Nurture Yourself. Turn off the TV, Listen to soft music, take a hot bath, go to the sauna, swimming & whirlpool. Have a relaxing and soothing massage, make a list of your goals and dream about it.
4. Make Changes in Your Diet. Eat all organic whole foods, eliminate all processed foods and refined foods from your diet.
5. Add Some Special Supplements Called Adaptogens. Holy Basil has been used to lower elevated cortisol levels and regulate blood sugar. Ashwagandha has been known to increase energy and mental alertness during the day. Research shows that it helps you sleep better at night.
6. Be Sure You Retain Lots of Vitamins and Minerals. Eat a variety of vegetables and fruits that contain lots of vitamins, minerals and fiber. And take some supplements.

VII. An Overactive Thyroid Can Also Cause Chronic Insomnia

An overactive thyroid can also cause chronic insomnia. In order to treat your chronic insomnia, you should also check your thyroid by doing a blood test for TSH, Free T4 and Free T3. If these tests are not normal, you need to take thyroid medication and/or adjust the dosage of the thyroid medication or switch to another type of thyroid medication (Synthroid, Armour / Desiccated Thyroid / ERFA Thyroid Tabs, Cytomel or other).

VIII. How to Fall Asleep in Less Than 30 Seconds, Posted by Steve Pavlina, July 10, 2013 [44]

Even a small cup of coffee in the morning can disrupt your ability to fall asleep quickly at night. You may also sleep less restfully, and you'll be prone to awaken more often throughout the night. Consequently, you may wake up tired and need extra sleep.

Simply eliminating all caffeine from your diet can improve your sleep habits tremendously. So if you haven't already done that, please do that first before you attempt the training method I explain later in this article. I also advise that you drop chocolate. The complete article can be found by clicking on the link in Reference # 44.

CAFFEINE CAUSES MUSCLE TENSION, CHRONIC PAIN & FATIGUE

I. Caffeine Disrupts Sleep and Causes Chronic Pain, Posted by A Massage Therapst Mr. Jordan Rothstein CMT [45]

After seeing many clients suffering from increased muscle tension and pain, massage therapist Mr. Jordan Rothstein CMT came to believe that, caffeine not only disrupts sleep but also causes pain. He posted the following information on his website:

Relationship Between Caffeine & Pain: There is a strong correlation between caffeine and pain. Caffeine makes the body's muscles tense, including the involuntary muscles in the internal organs. Prolonged consumption of caffeine in uncontrolled amounts could lead to muscle tension. Increased muscle tension overtime leads to the pain.

Caffeine plants also contain two other similar substances called theobromine and theophylline. These three substances caffeine, theobromine and theophylline belong to the same group of chemicals called methylxanthine alkaloids, which are drugs and central nervous system stimulants. These drugs are also toxic and addictive. If consumed excessively, they create a generalized stress in your body and make your muscles tense. High levels of muscle tension causes pain and over time it could lead to chronic pain.

Caffeine Disrupts Sleep: EEG (electroencephalography) tests in sleep labs showed that even one cup of coffee in the morning diminishes your sleep quality at night. So you wake up in the morning tired, dissatisfied with your sleep and tend to take naps in the afternoon. You will be tempted to consume another cup of coffee late in the afternoon as you feel drowsy due to lack of sleep the previous night. This vicious cycle continues like a chain reaction. That means you are addicted to caffeine and not sleeping well.

It was also proved in sleep labs that caffeine reduces REM sleep (Rapid Eye Movement). This means less dreams, less chance for recharging your mind. As a result, you become depressed. Caffeine also reduces or eliminates the deepest sleep possible in alpha and delta stages of sleep. This means less chance for recharging your body, less recovery from physical stress, less benefit from exercise, and less HGH (Human Growth Hormone) release. Lack of deep sleep is closely associated with two chronic pain conditions such as Fibromyalgia Syndrome (FMS) and Chronic Immune Deficiency Syndrome (CIDS).

Caffeine Increases Stress Reactions and Emotional Tension: Caffeine may exaggerate sympathetic adrenal-medullary responses to stressful events. Caffeine consumption causes repeated daily blood pressure elevation and increases stress reactivity, which could contribute to an increased risk of coronary heart disease.

Chocolate is a Stronger Pain Inducer than Caffeine: Chocolate is a stronger pain-inducer than coffee or tea. Chocolate causes dramatic increases in muscle tension and pain. Chocolate contains less caffeine than coffee, but it also contains theobromine and theophylline. If you drink coffee or tea and eat chocolate every day, the combined effect of caffeine, theobromine and theophylline could tense muscles and could cause chronic pain.

Quitting Caffeine Can Reduce Your Pain, and Sometimes Eliminate Pain:
People who have quit caffeine told the massage therapist Mr. Jordan Rothstein CMT that they had less pain, less anxiety, less anger, and felt less stressed. It may take a month or two to recover from withdrawal effects "drowsiness & fatigue" after quitting caffeine.

II. Caffeine Weakens the Adrenals and Leads to Chronic Back Pain, Posted by Sarah, Updated: March 19, 2017, Healthy Living [46]

The habit of prolonged consumption of caffeine weakens not only the adrenal glands but the entire area around them which includes the lower back. It is important to keep the adrenals healthy or weak adrenals can suck vital nutrients away from the ligaments and tendons. Ligaments bind bone to bone and tendons bind muscle to bone. The most important ligament is the one that joins and keeps the sacroiliac joint (SI Joint) firm, which is located at the lower back or pelvic area and which supports the weight of the entire body. When you overconsume caffeine, healthy nutrients do not enter the ligaments and tendons, so they get weak over time. As a result you develop the SI Joint and lower back pain. It would be wiser to end the caffeine addiction once and for all, and give your adrenals some relief, and strengthen those tendons and ligaments so that your back won't hurt anymore. Quitting the consumption of caffeine-containing foods and drinks could save your adrenals from serious predicaments.

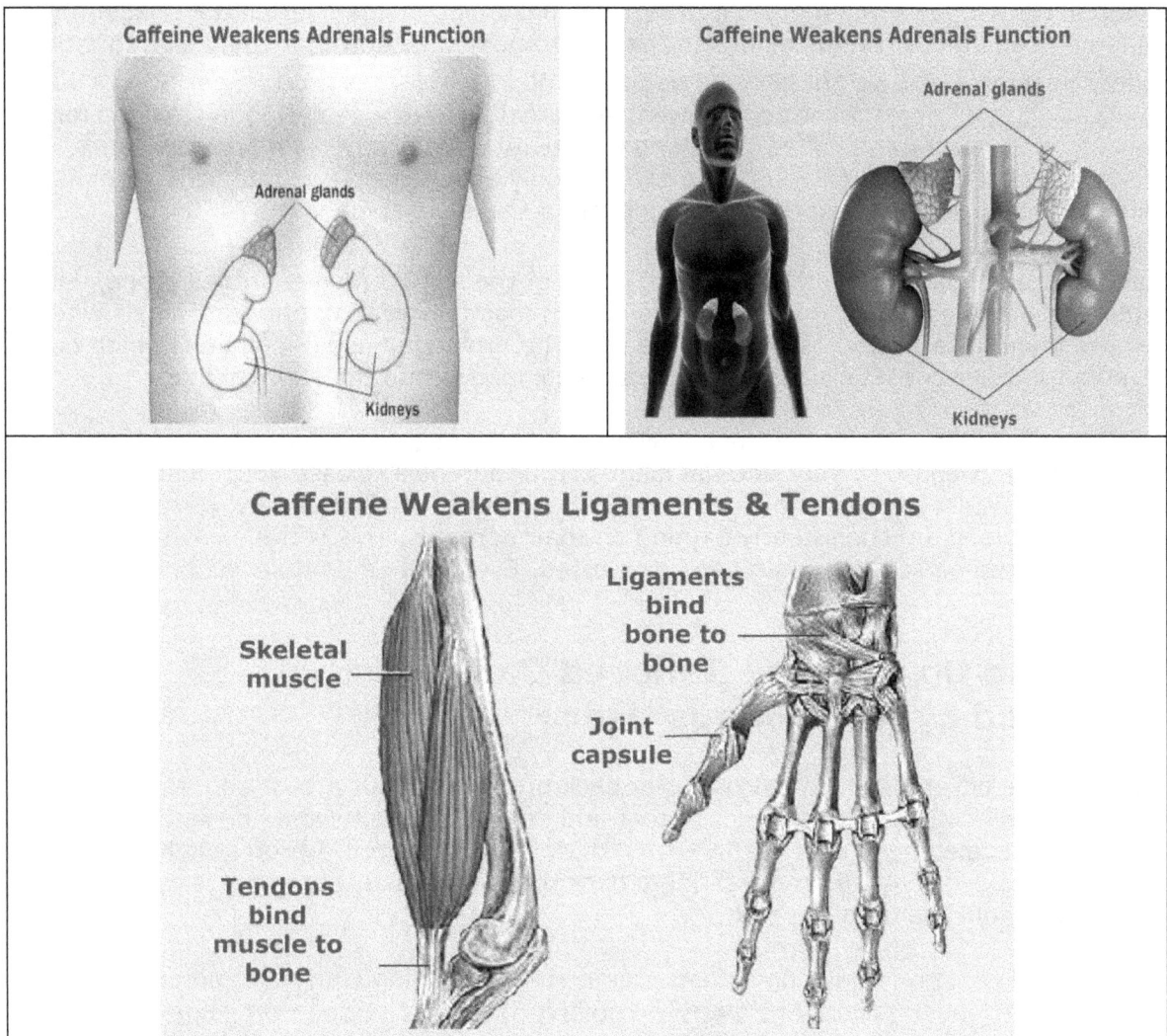

Figure 7.3 Caffeine weakens adrenals, ligaments and tendons.

III. Caffeine Effects on the Adrenal Function, Posted by Janice Skelton [47]

Daily consumption of caffeine stimulates neuron activity in the brain. Each time you drink a cup of coffee, neurons send messages to your pituitary gland which in turn alerts your adrenal glands to pump out adrenaline and cortisol. Adrenal glands function to produce hormones essential to life. The adrenal medulla is the inner portion of the adrenal gland, and produces adrenaline and noradrenaline. The adrenal cortex is the outer portion of the adrenal gland, and produces cortisol, estrogen, progesterone and testosterone. Adrenaline, noradrenaline, and cortisol are called stress hormones. High cortisol level then elevates heart rate and blood pressure, readying the body for a "fight or flight" response. Once the adrenals are provoked to release cortisol in such a manner over and over again by drinking coffee, a decreased resistance to stress occurs.

Caffeine puts the nervous and hormonal systems into a constant state of "fight or flight" stress response, depleting energy reserves. By consuming coffee over and over again, you would be pushing the adrenal glands to their extremes, an action that could lead to fatigue, anxiety, insomnia and weight gain. In addition, the liver releases more sugar to give you a temporary energy boost followed by low sugars or sugar-crash, resulting in cravings for simple carbohydrates and coffee. This kind of activity creates stress on adrenal glands, causing adrenal burnout. Therefore the caffeine only allows people to feel better temporarily while continuing to deplete the healthy function of the adrenal glands.

Healthy adrenal glands maintain adequate levels of the sex hormones progesterone, testosterone and estrogen. Adrenal glands cannot maintain healthy hormone levels when they are under attack by constant caffeine use. The prolonged use of caffeine in high doses elevates the cortisone levels and place the adrenal glands into the survival mode.

BuyTheDietSolution.com posted the following information: Last but not least, the caffeine in coffee and tea is abuse to your adrenal glands. Your adrenals release your "fight or flight" hormones basically giving you a nice "boost" when needed. Unfortunately, people who drink coffee all day long are consistently beating on their adrenals. This is the equivalent of whipping a tired horse even when he is exhausted. Eventually the horse will not move at all.

IV. Giving Up Caffeine Relieved Back Pain Posted by Anonymous User [48]

I am 42 years old and started having lower back problems about a year ago. My job is pretty physical, so I just attributed it to that and stress. The pain would be really bad in the morning and sometimes I'd have "flare-ups" during the day. Well, I tried switching mattresses, taking NSAIDS, and wearing a back brace before deciding that it was just something I would have to live with.

For unrelated reasons, I gave up caffeine completely (including chocolate, unfortunately). Incredibly, my back pain went away! I couldn't believe it. I hope that some of you can benefit from my experience. Yes, it's hard to give up that morning cup of coffee, but let me tell you, it's worth it! Just give it a try. It was only a few days after quitting caffeine completely that I had relief. Best of luck to everyone out there.

V. Coffee Can Create Joint Pain And Body Stiffness, Posted by Dr. Grady A. Deal, Ph.D., D.C [49]

Mostly neck pain, back pain and joint stiffness are caused by unhealthy lifestyles and underlying thyroid dysfunction. I have found in my holistic practice that the number one common cause of body stiffness from neck, back and joint stiffness, also including arm, elbow, hand, leg, knee and foot problems and also including exacerbation of chronic fibromyalgia pain are all mostly caused by bad habits such as: slouching during the waking hours, sleeping on the abdomen, sleeping with the arms and hands above the shoulders, sleeping on the same side or painful side most of the time, and sleeping in a twisted position that interferes with the blood and nerve circulation to the muscles and joints that cause stiffness and pain. The number two cause is diet and lifestyle related toxicity caused by unhealthy foods, milk, cheese, ice cream, **chocolate, MSG, coffee**, wine, beer, alcohol, cigarettes, street drugs, medications and anything that poisons the body that stresses, irritates and spasms skeletal muscles that pull the neck, back and joints out of alignment and fixate them causing joint stiffness and pain. Recent Finnish studies also directly linked coffee and joint pain. The number three cause is low thyroid function indicated by a basal resting temperature below 98.2°F that does not allow the needed warming effect of muscles and connective tissue that leads to joint stiffness and pain.

VI. Can Coffee Be Bad For Your Back? Posted by CureJoy Editorial [50]

Whether it is stress, inflammation, sleep disorders, or anxiety, your coffee could be making these conditions worse resulting in the aching back. In addition, coffee can intensify and aggravate your arthritis pain. According to Ayurvedic doctors, lower back pain is largely a problem of vata dosha and requires the person to cut out any inflammation-causing foods and stimulants such as coffee.

CAFFEINE ELEVATES CORTOSOL LEVELS AND CAUSES BACK PAIN:
It comes as no surprise that caffeine is a stimulant and kicks your body into high gear with heightened stress levels. This action drives the body's adrenal glands to work harder. A morning cup of coffee can keep your cortisol levels elevated all day long. In this "fight or flight" mode (fight or flight means the instinctive physiological response to a threatening situation, which readies one either to resist forcibly or to run away), your body is on the edge as it prepares for a possible attack. Whenever your muscles tense up, your sciatic nerve could get irritated, resulting in back pain.

CAFFEINE LINKED TO INSOMNIA & LOWER BACK PAIN: Those who consume multiple cups of coffee throughout the day, without thinking about the negative effects of caffeine, usually toss and turn too much while sleeping in the night and suffer tremendously from sleep deprivation and insomnia. Even if you consume coffee 6 hours prior to going to bed, sleep disturbances are likely to occur. According to many research studies, if you are not sleeping well, and not going into deep sleep or REM sleep every night, your risk of developing lower back pain is high. One study of adolescents found that not getting adequate sleep when they were 16 was a predictor of lower back pain, in boys as well as in girls.

CAFFEINE WITHDRAWAL COULD DEVELOP BACK PAIN TOO: If you decide to suddenly quit coffee and all caffeine-containing foods and drinks, you may do so but for a few days the withdrawal symptoms of the stimulant caffeine could be devastating. Each person reacts differently. For the first 24 hours, you may face headache, drowsiness and fatigue due to the absence of energy boost from coffee. You may also experience joint pain and overall muscular stiffness typically on the neck and shoulders. The pain could radiate to the other parts of the body, and you could experience severe back pain as well. Withdrawal symptoms tend to be worst between 20 hours and 51 hours and will usually last no longer than 9 days.

VII. Is Coffee Causing Those Aching Joints and Rheumatoid Arthritis? Posted by Dr. Ian Smith, July 26, 2000 [51]

Finnish researchers conducted two separate studies, both examining whether coffee had any association with the development of rheumatoid arthritis (RA). In the larger study of more than 18,000 participants, researchers found that drinking 11 or more cups of coffee a day increased the risk for developing the rheumatoid factor (RF), an antibody in the blood that doesn't necessarily cause RA but is believed to precede it by a few years. As many as 80 percent of the 2.1 million American patients suffering from RA test positive for this factor, convincing doctors that there is a significant association between the two.

In the second study of almost 7,000 participants, researchers found that those consuming four or more cups of coffee per day were two times more likely to develop rheumatoid arthritis (RA) than those who drank less. Because there are many types of arthritis, it is important to note that this RA was the type whose onset was associated with positive tests for rheumatoid factor.

VIII. Symptoms of Too Much Caffeine Posted by Teeccino Herbal Coffee [52]

Many people drink coffee, cup after cup, in an attempt to increase their energy by another hit of caffeine. Instead of feeling more energized, they start to experience energy crashes and find they cannot get off the caffeine roller coaster.

Excessive caffeine consumption causes muscular pain and tension including neck and back pain. If you suspect you are caffeine-sensitive, the best test is to completely eliminate caffeine from your diet, and avoid caffeinated beverages and coffee-flavored foods. Quit drinking coffee completely, and take Teeccino Herbal Coffee instead, which has zero caffeine in it.

IX. How I Quit Coffee Cold Turkey, Posted by Brandon [53]

After having drunk caffeine for so many years, Brandon has been experiencing upper middle back pain. When the pain became severe, Brandon decided to quit coffee expecting that his back pain would be relieved. His expectations have become a reality, as he no longer suffers from back pain. He has listed his entire experience on how he coped with the withdrawal symptoms after quitting coffee. The withdrawal symptoms were serious during the first 7 days, but with high willpower and self-discipline, he achieved his freedom from pain. He has detailed his entire experience on his webpage.

After living 21 days without coffee, Brandon experienced the following successful results:

◆ No headaches anymore
◆ More importantly, no tension in his upper middle back (back pain was gone)
◆ Improved concentration levels
◆ He is sleeping better and feeling more alert in the morning.
◆ He is having more regular and healthy bowel movements.
◆ Can now fall asleep by 11PM instead of 1AM which was when he was drinking coffee
◆ Increased awareness of the messages his body is sending. For example, he is feeling hungry at normal times (breakfast, lunch and dinner). No more cravings!
◆ Became more patient or relaxed while making decisions

CAFFEINE BLUES: WAKE UP TO THE HIDDEN DANGERS OF AMERICA'S #1 DRUG, Book Author: Stephen Cherniske, MS [2, 54, 55]

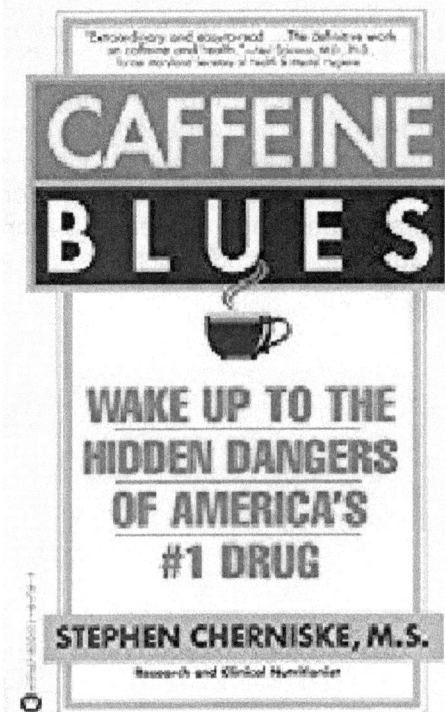

If you are a regular coffee drinker, and have been experiencing negative caffeine effects and caffeine-overdose symptoms, and want to take action, you should first read the aforementioned book "CAFFEINE BLUES". In this book, the author Stephen Cherniske describes all kinds of negative effects caused by caffeine, with references to many scientific research publications in Journals.

This book extensively details the way caffeine found in coffee, many teas, including green tea, chocolate, soft drinks and medications systematically breaks your health down. It is an extensive piece of work by a nutritionist, Stephen Cherniske, and extends to 451 pages of analysis of caffeine's hidden dangers.

FRONT COVER, CAFFEINE BLUES
♦Caffeine can't provide energy, only chemical stimulation, an induced emergency state that can lead to irritability, mood swings, and panic attacks.
♦ Caffeine's ultimate mood effect can be letdown, which can lead to depression and chronic fatigue.
♦ Caffeine gives the illusion of heightened alertness by dilating pupils, quickening heart rate and raising blood pressure. In fact, caffeine does not increase overall mental activity.

BACK COVER, CAFFEINE BLUES
Nearly 80 percent of all Americans - even doctors and journalists - are hooked on caffeine, this country's #1 addiction. A natural component of coffee, tea and chocolate - and added to drugs, soft drinks, candy and many other products, this powerful drug can affect brain function, hormone balance, and sleep patterns, while increasing your risk of osteoporosis, diabetes, ulcers, PMS, stroke, heart disease and certain types of cancer. Now for the first time, one of the most accomplished nutritional biochemists and medical writers in his field reveals the truth about caffeine and helps you kick the habit forever.

BY READING THE "CAFFEINE BLUES" BOOK, DISCOVER

♦ A step-by-step, clinically-proven program that reduces your caffeine intake without the headaches, fatigue and depression associated with withdrawal
♦ Effective ways to boost your energy with a group of newly-discovered nutrients, healthy beverages, better sleep and high-energy habits
♦ A fabulous new life of vibrant health, vitality and mental clarity

CHAPTER 1 COFFEE AND CAFFEINE: A Dose Of Reality

We have seen several well-marked cases of coffee excess. The sufferer is tremulous, and loses his self-command: He is the subject to fits of agitation and depression; he loses the color and has a haggard appearance. The appetite falls off, and symptoms of gastric catarrh may be manifested. The heart also suffers; it palpitates, or it intermits. As with other such agents, a renewed dose of the poison gives temporary relief, but at the cost of future misery. By miseries such as these, the best years of life may be spoilt.

The aforementioned paragraph was written by Sir T. Clifford Albutt and Dr. Walter Ernest Dixon, A System of Medicine, Volume II, London, 1909.

READ THROUGH THE FOLLOWING INFORMATION:
The following information was posted by Cheap Health Revolution [54]
(Copy and paste the URL onto your browser's address bar, and hit Enter key)
http://www.cheap-health-revolution.com/caffeine-blues.html

a. Caffeine & Hormones
http://www.cheap-health-revolution.com/caffeine-blues.html#chapter1

b. Benefits of Quitting Coffee
http://www.cheap-health-revolution.com/caffeine-blues.html#chapter2

c. Why Is Caffeine Harmful?
http://www.cheap-health-revolution.com/caffeine-blues.html#chapter3

d. Why Do I Like Caffeine?
http://www.cheap-health-revolution.com/caffeine-blues.html#chapter4

e. Vague Anxiety, Worries, Discomfort and Background Stress Caused by Caffeine
http://www.cheap-health-revolution.com/caffeine-blues.html#chapter5

f. How to Be Free of Caffeine and Restore Your Natural Energy Levels?
http://www.cheap-health-revolution.com/caffeine-blues.html#chapter6

g. The Hard Truth About Soft Drinks: Dangerous Levels of Caffeine and Sugar
http://www.cheap-health-revolution.com/caffeine-blues.html#chapter7

h. How Soon Can I Feel the Benefits of Quitting Caffeine?
http://www.cheap-health-revolution.com/caffeine-blues.html#chapter8

i. Politics of Coffee
http://www.cheap-health-revolution.com/caffeine-blues.html#chapter9

SOME IMPORTANT PARAGRAPHS OF THE BOOK "CAFFEINE BLUES:"

Caffeine is clearly addictive, completely unregulated, and its presence in our foods and beverages is often hidden! Almost daily I see a patient whose symptoms are made worse by the consumption of caffeine. The drug contributes to palpitations, panic attacks, hypoglycemia, gastritis, fatigue, insomnia, and PMS, to name a few. Some people are so sensitive to caffeine that they don't realize a fruit drink with hidden caffeine can cause their symptoms. Caffeine Blues by Stephen Cherniske MS, page xi, Foreword

Caffeine does not provide energy—only chemical stimulation. The perceived "energy" comes from the body's struggle to adapt to increased blood levels of stress hormones. In most cases, this induced emergency state leads to well-defined side effects collectively known as caffeinism. Ironically, caffeinism is characterized by fatigue. Caffeine Blues by Stephen Cherniske MS, page 6

Caffeinism and Chronic Fatigue: "Caffeinism" is a state of chronic toxicity resulting from excess caffeine consumption. Caffeinism usually combines physical addiction with a wide range of debilitating effects, most notably anxiety, irritability, mood swings, sleep disturbance, depression, and fatigue. Caffeine Blues by Stephen Cherniske MS, page 36

Tolerance: The body develops a tolerance for caffeine so that greater amounts are required to produce the same level of stimulation. Seventy-five percent of the caffeine-dependent group reported tolerance.
Caffeine Blues by Stephen Cherniske MS, page 42

Why is Caffeine Harmful? Caffeinism: It Could Happen to You! In over a decade of practice as a clinical nutritionist, I have seen firsthand, with thousands of clients, that caffeine is a health hazard. Anxiety, muscle aches, PMS (premenstrual syndrome), headaches, heartburn, insomnia, and irritability are the most common symptoms, and they can usually be lessened or eliminated simply by avoiding caffeine.
Caffeine Blues by Stephen Cherniske MS, page 42

On the physical level, we need a steady source of energy to accomplish our goals. Nothing is more frustrating than to be motivated, to have a great plan, but no energy to carry it out. When I ask patients about their reasons for drinking coffee, the most common response is: "I need the energy". The irony is that caffeine is a major cause of fatigue. Depending on caffeine to get you through the day might work for a while, but in the long run it will make your dreams harder and harder to achieve. Caffeine Blues by Stephen Cherniske MS, page 43

It doesn't take a genius to see that there might be a downside to all of this neuron activity. In fact, uncontrolled neuron firing creates an emergency situation, which triggers the pituitary gland in the brain to secrete ACTH (adrenocorticotrophic hormone). ACTH tells the adrenal glands to pump out stress hormones—the next major side effect of caffeine. Caffeine Blues by Stephen Cherniske MS, page 56

Caffeine also stimulates the production of norepinephrine, another stress hormone that acts directly on the brain and nervous system. Epinephrine and norepinephrine are responsible for increased heart rate, increased blood pressure, and that "emergency" feeling. In fact, the emergency is quite real. Caffeine can trigger a classic fight-or-flight stress reaction with all of the results listed in Illustration. Caffeine Blues by Stephen Cherniske MS, page 57
Caffeine causes adrenal exhaustion, i.e. the exhaustion of the adrenal glands. Adrenal exhaustion, in turn, has other consequences: "I was seeing patients every day with serious

health problems that strong, healthy adrenals could have prevented. Why were these people vulnerable to allergy, inflammation, hypertension, infection, and fatigue?"
Caffeine Blues by Stephen Cherniske MS, page 65

Research is revealing that cortisol and DHEA, both produced in the adrenal cortex, hold an inverse relationship. As serum cortisol increases, DHEA levels fall. It may be that stress and caffeine create such a high need for cortisol that the exhausted adrenals simply cannot maintain production of DHEA at optimal levels.
Caffeine Blues by Stephen Cherniske MS, page 68

Caffeine triggers a stress response that involves a surge in adrenal hormones and the classic fight-or-flight "emergency", affecting virtually every cell in the body.
Caffeine Blues by Stephen Cherniske MS, page 98

The second way that caffeine contributes to depression is, of course, the withdrawal reaction, the most prevalent symptoms being headache, depression, and fatigue. Three facts are important to grasp in regard to withdrawal. First of all, each of the symptoms compounds or magnifies the depressive effect. Secondly, withdrawal can occur even in light caffeine users. And third, withdrawal reactions can be evident even when caffeine is withheld for just a few hours. Some people feel depressed or anxious if they're simply late for their morning or afternoon cup. That's not only a powerful motivation to consume the beverage, but it also creates an often-unidentified source of background stress.
Caffeine Blues by Stephen Cherniske MS, page 112

Caffeine even in small doses, is a potent cerebral vasoconstrictor. One study illustrated that a dose of 250 g (15 Oz of coffee) produced approximately a 30% decrease in whole-brain cerebral blood flow (Referenced to scientific journal publication). This is not only unfortunate, it is dangerous, because at the same time, caffeine increases blood pressure in the brain, leading to an increased risk of stroke.
Caffeine Blues by Stephen Cherniske MS, page 122

A great many people are addicted to caffeine and abuse it without being aware of the consequences. Depending on individual sensitivity, as little as two cups of coffee per day has been shown to produce anxiety, insomnia, irritability, and dizziness.
Caffeine Blues by Stephen Cherniske MS, page 127

Although the phenomenon of caffeine withdrawal has been described previously, the present report documents that the incidence of caffeine withdrawal is higher (100 percent of subjects), the daily dose level at which withdrawal occurs is lower (roughly equivalent to the amount of caffeine in a single cup of strong brewed coffee or three cans of caffeinated soft drink), and the range of symptoms experienced is broader (including headache, fatigue and other dysphoric mood changes, muscle pain/stiffness, flu-like feelings, nausea/vomiting and craving for caffeine) than heretofore recognized.
Caffeine Blues by Stephen Cherniske MS, page 189

Recovery from fibromyalgia is unlikely as long as your adrenals are stressed. Avoiding caffeine will greatly increase your chance of recovery.
Caffeine Blues by Stephen Cherniske MS, page 212-213

Caffeine causes anxiety, which is part of the vicious cycle of stress and fatigue.
The next result is that inflammation and pain are intensified.
Caffeine Blues, by Stephen Cherniske MS, page 213
Men can significantly reduce their risk for urinary and prostate problems by getting off coffee and caffeine. Caffeine Blues by Stephen Cherniske MS, page 216

If it's a 'regular' cola, your body is jolted by about nine teaspoons of sugar. (When was the last time you put nine teaspoons of sugar in a beverage?) In response, your blood glucose levels rise quickly and your pancreas pour out insulin. Both the elevated glucose and insulin foster weight gain. If it's a diet cola, your brain registers the intense sweetness of aspartame and instructs the intestinal tract to prepare for an enormous intake of calories. Your body creates enzymes to convert future calories to fat, just like it did 10,000 years ago. So even through the beverage contains only one calorie (a concept your brain and body do not understand), you remain primed to create fat as soon as you eat some real food. That's why the more artificial sweeteners you consume, the more likely you are actually to gain weight - as confirmed by a study of 80,000 women over a period of six years."
Caffeine Blues by Stephen Cherniske MS, page 280

Soft drinks are implicated in reports of fatigue and sleep disturbance as well as coffee. A direct relationship was reported among caffeine intake, disturbed sleep, and reported tiredness during the day. Caffeine Blues by Stephen Cherniske MS, page 287

High-calorie soft drinks are implicated in weight gain among children.
Caffeine Blues by Stephen Cherniske MS, page 289

Soft drink intake is linked to a number of other conditions, including bone fractures due to deficient calcium, tooth decay, tooth tissue loss, and dehydration.
Caffeine Blues by Stephen Cherniske MS, page 289

Headache isn't the only side effect you may experience from quitting caffeine. It's just the most obvious. Your body, which has become accustomed to drug-induced stimulation, needs to recover its natural abundant energy supply. After all, most people consume caffeine to boost their energy levels, so restoring natural energy production once you're off the bean is critical. If you find yourself unable to muster the oomph to face the day, or crippled by "brain fog" that won't clear, you'll get discouraged quickly. Any program for quitting caffeine must provide a variety of successful methods to deal with fatigue so you don't go running back to caffeine. Caffeine Blues by Stephen Cherniske MS, page 336

Human body is designed to last about 120 years, and it is quite capable of sustaining a high level of energy until the very end. So why don't we feel this vigor and vitality? It's not because we lose it. We throw it away. We fall into the trap of sedentary living, poor diet, and caffeine. When we stop moving, we lose metabolic efficiency.
Caffeine Blues by Stephen Cherniske MS, page 339

To recover your natural energy, you must take three important steps: Eliminate caffeine abuse, boost your nutritional intake, and develop a habit of regular exercise. The order in which you take these steps is also very important. You need to restore your metabolic efficiency. You then take that renewed energy and use it to build up an exercise program that feels good and works. Caffeine Blues by Stephen Cherniske MS, page 339-340

You may find that after you quit caffeine, for a period of some time it seems like your body needs an unusual amount of sleep. If you allow yourself to benefit from increased sleep hours during your first few weeks off caffeine, your body will more rapidly complete the high level of repair necessary in your organs and nervous system. Caffeine Blues by Stephen Cherniske MS, page 369

MORE IMPORTANT PARAGRAPHS OF THE BOOK "CAFFEINE BLUES:"
More important paragraph of the book "Caffeine Blues can be found on the article posted by Dani Veracity titled "The hidden dangers of caffeine: How coffee causes exhaustion, fatigue and addiction". [56]

COFFEEINE CONSUMPTION GUIDELINES (by Dr. RK)

● **Limited caffeine consumption has positive effects**. Each person is different! So each person must determine optimum number of cups of coffee (how many cups of coffee per day) by trial and error, and must drink all that coffee before noon.

● **Overconsumption of caffeine disrupts sleep, causes chronic insomnia, chronic pain, fatigue and other health issues**. Anxiety, insomnia, muscle aches, PMS (premenstrual syndrome), headaches, heartburn, and irritability are the other common symptoms.

● You should always keep an eye on every food item and drink you consume in restaurants and coffee-shops, as most drinks and some foods contain caffeine. For example, Coke, Diet Coke, Pepsi, Diet Pepsi and other soft drinks contain a lot of caffeine. Beware of the foods and drinks that contain elevated levels of caffeine, and keep them in your block list. Be cautious about caffeine content whenever you eat and drink out.

● Please do not take coffee or decaf in restaurants as the caffeine content there could be dangerously high. For example, Americano is loaded with too much caffeine. Do your own research and drink coffee or decaf at home.

● Research and find out exactly how much caffeine is present per cup of that selected volume of coffee you aimed to drink. Know exactly how much caffeine you consume per day by doing some reasonable calculations and by checking the labels of the coffee you purchased. If you do so, you can easily control the amount of caffeine being consumed per day, and can take action if you are affected by overconsumption.

● If you are too sensitive to caffeine, more particularly if you are over 55 years old with underlying health conditions, you better make your coffee at home from organic ground coffee powder. Stick to the same brand, stick to the same schedule and plan ahead by consuming optimal number of cups of coffee (1 cup, 2 cups or 3 cups per day to be determined by trial and error).

● Under critical circumstances, quitting coffee would be a great idea at least for some time. You can always get back to consuming limited coffee again. Withdrawal symptoms would last a few days, and it is not that difficult to quit coffee drinking. Try it out, you quit coffee for some time and you can re-start it anytime if needed. For example if you are too sleepy during the day, you need to re-introduce coffee or decaf again to keep you alert. Your own research would guide you and help you cure your insomnia and save your life.

● **Instead of quitting coffee, you can consume "Decaf Coffee" to avoid withdrawal symptoms**.

♦ Please note that decaf is not 100% free of caffeine. The decaffeination process does not allow to remove more than 97% of the caffeine, meaning that at least 3% of caffeine is still present in decaf coffee (in some brands, it could be a lot more than 3% of caffeine).

♦ So "Decaf Coffee" presents an opportunity for you to consume a tiny or very limited amount of caffeine that could help keep you alert during the day. However consume all that decaf your body needs before noon, and do not consume any coffee or decaf after noon.

CAFFEINE ALTERNATIVES

All kinds of coffee and any regular tea, including green tea, contain caffeine. However herbal tea does not contain caffeine. The following products are available in many heath food stores as alternatives to coffee. All these products, also called herbal coffees, contain chicory, which has some adverse side effects. They don't taste as good as some people say. It is up to the each individual to try and find out if any of these products can be used as an alternative to coffee drinking. You can purchase the following products in a local health food store. You can also try to find them on Amazon or by doing Google search.

1. Teeccino Caffe, Inc
   Santa Barbara, CA-93140
   Toll Free: 1-800-493-3434
   http://teeccino.com/

2. ALKAVA
   7298 Hume Avenue,
   Delta, BC, Canada, V4G 1C5
   Ph: 604-946-7277
   https://www.londondrugs.com/

3. Dandy Blend
   P.O.Box 446
   Valley City, Ohio 44280
   http://www.dandyblend.com/

4. Pero All Natural Beverage Coffee Substitute
   1455 Broad Street, 4th Floor
   Bloomfield, NJ 07003
   Phone: 973-338-1499
   https://worldfiner.com/

5. Organic Rooibas Red Tea (Herbal Tea, Containing No Caffeine), preferably taken with organic skim milk or 1% milk. It is being recommended as the best alternative to coffee drinking. It tastes good, gives energy, and you would be easily accustomed to it within a week after quitting coffee. Try It Out!

ENJOY ROOIBOS TEA.

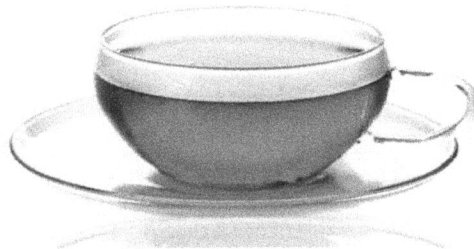

Figure 7.4 Rooibas red tea (100% certified organic herbal tea).

Rooibas Red Tea (100% Certified Organic Herbal Tea)
Best Caffeine Alternative (Milk Tea) Being Recommended!

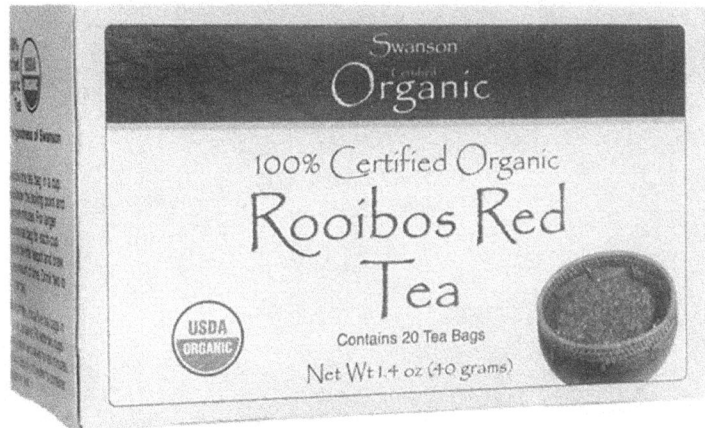

Courtesy of Swanson Vitamins
Rooibos Red Tea is available at www.swansonvitamins.com
Rooibos Red Tea (100% Certified Organic), Item # SWF082, 20 Bags, $3.99
https://www.swansonvitamins.com/swanson-organic-certified-organic-rooibos-red-tea-20-bags-s

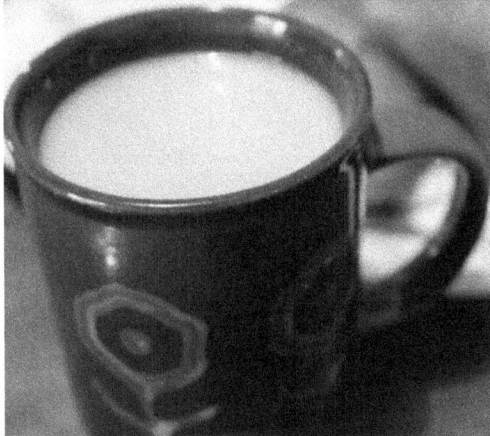

Rooibas Chai (Herbal Tea + Hot Water + Hot Milk + Cardamom)

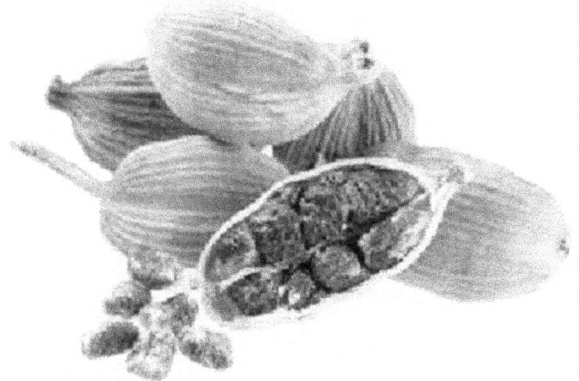

Cardamom Pods and Seeds

PREPARATION OF MILK HERBAL TEA/CHAI (Alternative to Coffee)

1. Boil purified water (do not drink tap water) using an electric kettle.
2. Add one-quarter cup of organic skim milk or 1% milk to a mug, and microwave it for 1 minute.
3. Place two or three bags of Organic Rooibas Red Tea/Ginger Tea/Other Organic Herbal Tea in the mug that contained one-quarter cup of hot organic skim milk or 1% milk.
4. Pour boiled water into the mug until it is full, and allow the tea from tea-bags to dissolve in the mug. You can press the tea bags to the wall of the mug by using a spoon. You will see the golden-brown color or chai color of herbal tea made from hot water and milk, as shown in the picture above.
5. Break cardamom pods with a knife and remove the seeds and add both skin and seeds to the hot tea in the mug, you will sense a delicious aroma and flavor while drinking the tea. Cardamom pods and seeds can be chewed as a breath freshener. Cardamom has many health benefits. Both the seeds and pod give a pleasant aroma and flavor. Enjoy the Chai!

Figure 7.5 Chai made from organic Rooibas red tea, hot water, hot milk & cardamom.

REFERENCES

HISTORY OF CAFFEEINE
1. A Secret History of Coffee, Cola & Cola, Written and Illustrated by Richard Cortes, ISBN # 978-1-61775-134-9, Published by Akashic Books, 2012.

2. Caffeine Blues: Wake Up to the Hidden Dangers of America's #1 Drug by Stephen Cherniske, MS, ISBN # 0446673919, Book Published by Warner Books, New York, 1998.

3. Caffeine (from Wikipedia)
https://en.wikipedia.org/wiki/Caffeine

SOURCES OF CAFFEINE
4. Sources of Caffeine, 2nd Page (click on right arrow), Posted by Coffee and Health.
https://www.coffeeandhealth.org/topic-overview/sources-of-caffeine/

5. Coffee and Health, Posted by Eufic.Org, Aug 6, 2007.
http://www.eufic.org/en/whats-in-food/article/caffeine-and-health

CAFFEINE CONSUMPTION GUIDELINES
6. Caffeine Content in Foods & Drinks, FDA Website.
https://www.fda.gov/downloads/ucm200805.pdf

7. Caffeine in Food, Health Canada.
http://www.hc-sc.gc.ca/fn-an/securit/addit/caf/food-caf-aliments-eng.php

8. What is Caffeine? Is It Bad for My Health? Dietitians of Canada, March 25, 2013.
https://www.dietitians.ca/Your-Health/Nutrition-A-Z/Caffeine/What-is-Caffeine-.aspx

9. Natural T Side Effects, Posted by WhatGo.
http://effectchoices.blogspot.ca/2017/04/natural-t-side-effects.html

CAFFEINE CONSUMPTION: HOW MUCH IS TOO MUCH?
10. This is how much caffeine it takes to kill an average person, Mary Bowerman, USA TODAY Network Published 8:22 a.m. ET May 16, 2017 | Updated 3:27 p.m. ET May 16, 2017.
https://www.usatoday.com/story/news/nation-now/2017/05/16/south-carolina-teen-dies-caffeine-how-much-coffee-can-kill-you/99975022/

CAFFEINE CONTENT IN FOODS & DRINKS
11. Caffeine Content in Foods and Drinks Varies Significantly and Cannot Be Trusted, Sleep and Caffeine, Sleep Education.
http://www.sleepeducation.org/news/2013/08/01/sleep-and-caffeine

12. Sources of Caffeine in Commonly Consumed Beverages, Posted by Coffee and Health.
https://www.coffeeandhealth.org/topic-overview/sources-of-caffeine-infographic/

13. How Much Caffeine is Present in A Standard Serrving?, Posted by Health Navigator.
https://www.healthnavigator.org.nz/healthy-living/eating-drinking/c/caffeine/?tab=12422

14. How Much Caffeine in Your Drinks, Posted by Love ThisPic.
http://www.lovethispic.com/image/178241/how-much-caffeine-in-your-drinks

LIMITED CAFFEINE CONSUMPTION HAS POSITIVE EFFECTS
15. Caffeine Myths & Facts, WebMD.
http://www.webmd.com/diet/caffeine-myths-and-facts#1
http://www.webmd.com/diet/caffeine-myths-and-facts

UNBELIEVABLE FACTS ABOUT CAFFEINE
16. 7 Unbelievable Facts About Caffeine.
https://healthprep.com/featured/7-unbelievable-facts-about-what-caffeine-does-to-your-body/

POSITIVE AND NEGATIVE EFFECTS OF CAFFEINE
17. The Harmful Effects of Overdosing on Coffee, Pros & Cons of Coffee Consumption by James Tang.
https://www.acetutors.com.sg/The-Harmful-Effects-of-Overdosing-on-Coffee

18. Caffeine – how bad is it for you? by hellomagazine.com, June 21, 2012.
https://ca.hellomagazine.com/healthandbeauty/health-and-fitness/201206218417/caffeine-effects-body/

19. Caffeine Intake- Positive and Negative Effects on Health by Theravive, June 19, 2014.
https://www.theravive.com/today/post/caffeine-intake-positive-and-negative-effects-on-health-0001513.aspx

CAFFEINE OVERDOSE SYMPTOMS
20. Caffeine from Wikipedia.
https://en.wikipedia.org/wiki/Caffeine

21. Caffeine Overdose Symptoms.
https://en.wikipedia.org/wiki/Caffeine#/media/File:Main_symptoms_of_Caffeine_overdose.svg

22. Caffeine is More Like an Illegal Drug Than You Realized by Dylan Moore August 31, 2017.
http://www.toptenz.net/caffeine-like-illegal-drug-realized.php

23. Are You At Risk of Cafei8ne Overdose?, Guest post from blogger Robert Milton who blogs for Jollyville Dental, an Austin dentist, who specializes in cosmetic dental procedures and Invisalign braces.
http://www.promotehealth.info/are-you-at-risk-of-a-caffeine-overdose/

24. Main Symptoms of Caffeine Overdose, WP Clipart, Medical Problems.
https://www.wpclipart.com/medical/medical_problems/drugs/caffeine/Caffeine_overdose_symptoms.png.html

CAFFEINE IS DANGEROUS
25. Documented Deaths By Caffeine, Posted by Caffeine Informer Staff.
https://www.caffeineinformer.com/a-real-life-death-by-caffeine

26. A 16-Year-Old Student in South Carolina Died, Posted by Buzz Feed News, May 16, 2017.
https://www.buzzfeed.com/tasneemnashrulla/a-teenager-died-of-a-caffeine-overdose?utm_term=.yux0kXEBP#.ohdpr1XOB

WHY CAFFEINE IS ADDICTIVE?
27. Mitchell Moffit and Gregory Brown demystify the inner workings of caffeine in their latest ASAP Science video. Watch the animation on the video to understand how caffeine molecules replace adenosine molecules in the receptors of your brain to make you alert and to become addictive.

YouTube Video: Your Brain On Coffee.
https://www.youtube.com/watch?v=4YOwEqGykDM

28. Here is what coffee actually does to your brain (That damn adenosine).
Watch the animation on the video to understand how caffeine molecules replace adenosine molecules in the brain to become addictive, TheJournal.ie of Ireland. Sept 7th, 2014.
http://www.thejournal.ie/coffee-brain-1648663-Sep2014/

29. Here Is What Coffee Actually Does To Your Brain, Lauren F Friedman, Aug. 28, 2014. Watch the animation on the website to understand how caffeine molecules replace adenosine molecules.
http://www.businessinsider.com/how-does-coffee-affect-your-brain-2014-8

30. Review Posted by Tobeagenius on Coffee Addiction.
http://thearialligraphyproject.tumblr.com/post/136800255812/littlestudysession-tobeagenius-coffee

31. This Is How Your Brain Becomes Addicted To Caffeine by Joseph Stromberg, smithsonian.com, August 9, 2013.
https://www.smithsonianmag.com/science-nature/this-is-how-your-brain-becomes-addicted-to-caffeine-26861037/

https://www.smithsonianmag.com/science-nature/this-is-how-your-brain-becomes-addicted-to-caffeine-26861037/?no-ist

32. Does Caffeine Give You Energy? The Truth About Caffeine Fatigue, Posted by Ari Whitten, The Energy Blue Print.
https://www.theenergyblueprint.com/caffeine-fatigue/

33. How Caffeine Works (Caffeine, Adenosine, Adrenaline) by Marshall Brain, Charles W Bryant & Matt Cunningham, How Stuff Works.
http://science.howstuffworks.com/caffeine4.htm

34. Caffeine: The Silent Killer of Success by Travis Bradberry, August 21, 2012, Forbes.com.
https://www.forbes.com/sites/travisbradberry/2012/08/21/caffeine-the-silent-killer-of-emotional-intelligence/#37cb90e118ce

35. The Effects of Caffeine on Adenosine by Helen Anderson, Last Updated: Oct 03, 2017.
http://www.livestrong.com/article/481979-the-effects-of-caffeine-on-adenosine/

36. What Caffeine Really Does to Your Brain? Posted by David DiSalvo, health Contributor.
https://www.forbes.com/sites/daviddisalvo/2012/07/26/what-caffeine-really-does-to-your-brain/#f3e57f048b67

37. Open for Discussion: Caffeine, Caffeine in the Brain, by Barbara Sitzman and Regis Goode, October 2013.
https://www.acs.org/content/acs/en/education/resources/highschool/chemmatters/past-issues/archive-2013-2014/caffeine.html

CAFFEINE CAUSES SLEEP DISTURBANCES & INSOMNIA
JOURNAL PUBLICATIONS

38. Caffeine Effects on Sleep Taken 0, 3, or 6 Hours before Going to Bed, by Christopher Drake, Ph.D., F.A.A.S.M., Timothy Roehrs, Ph.D., F.A.A.S.M. John Shambroom, B.S. Thomas Roth, Ph.D, Journal of Clinical Sleep Medicine.
http://www.aasmnet.org/jcsm/ViewAbstract.aspx?pid=29198

39. Effect of caffeine on sleep EEG study in late middle age people, VLASTA BREZINOVA, Sleep Laboratory, Department of Psychiatry, University of Edinburgh, Edinburgh, EH105HF, Scotland. Journal Reference: Br. J. Clin. Pharmac. (1974), 1, 203-208.
https://www.ncbi.nlm.nih.gov/pmc/articles/PMC1402564/

Complete Article.
https://www.ncbi.nlm.nih.gov/pmc/articles/PMC1402564/pdf/brjclinpharm00282-0023.pdf

40. Even Afternoon Coffee Disrupts Sleep, Study Finds, Posted by NHS Choices of the Government UK, 2013.
http://www.nhs.uk/news/2013/11November/Pages/Even-afternoon-coffee-disrupts-sleep-study-finds.aspx

41. Caffeine-Induced Sleep Disorder (from Wikipedia).
https://en.wikipedia.org/wiki/Caffeine-induced_sleep_disorder

42. Cortisol Levels – How Caffeine Intake Affects Stress Hormones by Diane Mohlman.
http://www.shapefit.com/diet/cortisol-caffeine.html

43. Want to Sleep Better? First, Reduce Your Cortisol Levels Then Follow These Six Key Tips, Posted by Body-Ecology.
https://bodyecology.com/articles/reduce_your_cortisol_levels.php

44. How to Fall Asleep in Less Than 30 Seconds? Posted by Steve Pavlina, July 10, 2013.
https://www.stevepavlina.com/blog/2013/07/how-to-fall-asleep-in-less-than-30-seconds/

CAFFEINE CAUSES MUSCLE TENSION, PAIN & FATIGUE

45. Caffeine: Cup of Pain, Liquid Stress, Posted by Jordan Rothstein CMT.
http://bodytechnician.com/caffeine.html

46. Is Caffeine Causing Your Chronic Back Pain? Posted by Sarah, March 19, 2017.
https://www.thehealthyhomeeconomist.com/is-caffeine-causing-your-back-pain/

47. Caffeine Effects on the Adrenal Function Posted by Janice Skelton, Sep 17, 2011.
http://www.livestrong.com/article/269199-caffeine-effects-on-the-adrenal-function/

48. Giving Up Caffeine Helped Me!, Posted by Anonymous User, May 27, 2009.
https://www.spine-health.com/forum/discussion/21618/pain/lower-back-pain/giving-caffeine-helped-me

49. Coffee Can Create Joint Pain And Body Stiffness, Posted by Dr. Grady A. Deal, Ph.D., D.C.
https://www.bodyzone.com/most-neck-back-and-joint-stiffness-and-pain-are-caused-by-unhealthy-lifestyles-and-underlying-thyroid-dysfunction/

50. Can Coffee Be Bad For Your Back?, Posted by CureJoy Editorial, Feb 7, 2017.
https://www.curejoy.com/content/can-coffee-cause-backpain/

51. Is Coffee Causing Those Aching Joints? by Dr. Ian Smith, July 26, 2000.
http://content.time.com/time/magazine/article/0,9171,50955,00.html

52. Symptoms of Too Much Caffeine by Teeccino (Herbal Coffee).
http://teeccino.com/building_optimal_health/128/Symptoms-of-Too-Much-Caffeine.html

53. How I quit coffee cold turkey & the first 7 days without caffeine (hint: it sucked)
Posted by Brandon on January 15, 2014 in Healthy Habits, Lifestyle, Travel.
http://www.theyoganomads.com/survive-5-year-coffee-addiction-expect-first-7-days-hint-sucked/

CAFFEINE BLUES BOOK

54. Caffeine Blues: Wake Up to the Hidden Dangers of America's #1 Drug, Review Posted by Cheap Health Revolution.
http://www.cheap-health-revolution.com/caffeine-blues.html

55. CAFFEINE BLUES (BOOK) IS AVAILABLE ONLINE (First Few Pages).
https://www.scribd.com/doc/225997000/Caffeine-Blues

56. The hidden dangers of caffeine: How coffee causes exhaustion, fatigue and addiction, Review Posted by Dani Veracity, October 11, 2005.
http://www.naturalnews.com/012352_caffeine_coffee.html

P.S.: For the Digital Book, if the links don't work, please copy and paste the URL onto your browser's address bar, and hit the Enter key.

About the Author

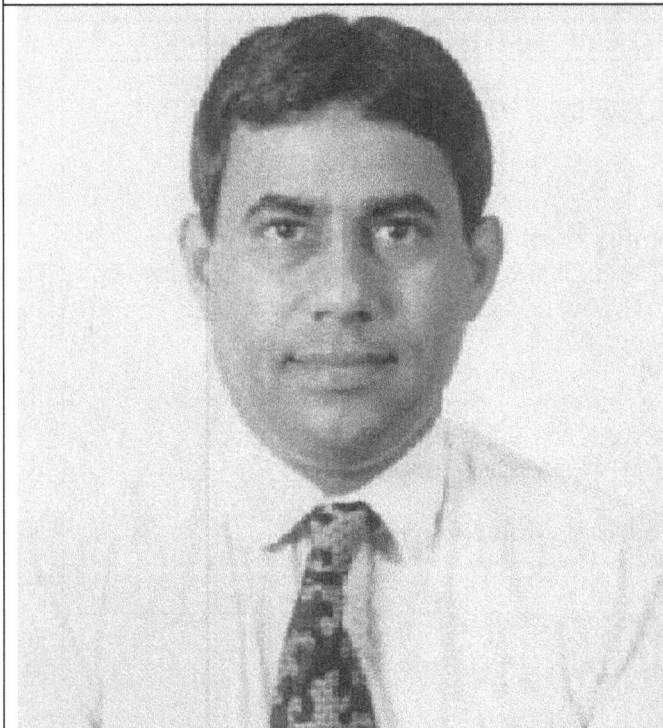

Dr. Rao M Konduru was a Chemical Engineer, and held two Master's degrees and two doctorates and two post-doctoral titles, all in chemical engineering. He published a book in 2003 titled "Permanent Diabetes Control," which earned immense respect and appreciation. Many people said it was a wonderful book. After suffering from a sudden heart attack in 1998, even though his left artery was 75% clogged with severe angina, he said "NO" to bypass surgery. He did what none of us would even think of doing. He simply relied on his natural self-prevention diet and exercise, and with it he reversed his critical diabetic heart disease in a matter of months, and developed a method to accomplish Permanent Diabetes Control. He also came up with a trial-and-error procedure to determine the optimal insulin dose that would tightly control diabetes, and would allow a diabetic person to live like a normal person for the rest of his/her life.

Dr. Rao M Konduru maintained his hemoglobin A1c level under 6.0% consistently. His personal best hemoglobin A1c level of 5.0% was an extraordinary result any diabetic person would hope to accomplish in a lifetime. Perhaps Dr. Rao M Konduru was the only diabetic person lived in this world with "Permanent Diabetes Control".

Once again, health demons such as uncontrollable weight gain, sleep apnea and chronic insomnia came his way. He did not give up, but persisted on discovering new, natural and effortless treatments of his own in reversing these most difficult disorders. His extensive scientific research experience and his powerful knowledge helped him battle and combat these life challenges. He figured out their root causes, and developed natural yet powerful techniques to cure these health disorders himself. After losing 40 pounds of weight and 12 inches around the waist, he successfully reversed his obesity, obstructive sleep apnea and chronic insomnia. He carefully created and published the following excellent guidebooks on Amazon so that others can benefit and be inspired to achieve similar results. His most recent book "Drinking Water Guide" is a 540-page book of wealth of information on drinking water for the rest of us.

1. Permanent Diabetes Control — www.mydiabetescontrol.com
2. The Secret to Controlling Type 2 Diabetes — www.mydiabetescontrol.com
3. Reversing Obesity — www.reversingsleepapnea.com/ebook2.html
4. Reversing Sleep Apnea — www.reversingsleepapnea.com
5. Reversing Insomnia — www.reversinginsomnia.com
6. Reversing Insomnia in 3 Days — www.reversinginsomnia.com
7. Drinking Water Guide — www.drinkingwaterguide.com
8. Drinking Water Guide-II — www.drinkingwaterguide.com
9. The Origin of the Earth's Water — www.drinkingwaterguide.com
10. Autobiography Of Dr. Rao M Konduru — www.mydiabetescontrol.com/Bio/
- Prime Publishing Co.

PLEASE WRITE A REVIEW ABOUT THIS BOOK

Now that you have read this book, please write a review about this book, and post your review on Amazon.

a. Please log into your Amazon account,
b. Search for this book "Reversing Insomnia, Author: Rao Konduru, PhD",
   or by using ISBN # 9780973112016, and click on the book cover & scroll down,
c. Click on "Customer Reviews", click on "Write a customer review" button,
   and "Create Review" box pops up.
d. Kindly write your REVIEW in the Write-Your-Review box, type a Headline,
   and click on 5 stars overall rating (you can give up to 5 stars).
e. Click on "Submit" button, and your review will be registered on Amazon.
f. Amazon will acknowledge your review with an email confirmation!

Thanks for posting your review!
Your opinion counts!

YOUR OPINION
COUNTS!

Kindle eBook Is Available on Amazon

You can read this book on your computer, laptop, tablet, e-reader, iPhone, or any Kindle device by purchasing Kindle eBook. It is available on Amazon.
Please log into your Amazon account, and search for "Reversing Insomnia, Kindle eBook" or by using ASIN # B07L2347F9.

The end of the book "Reversing Insomnia".

BEST WISHES!

www.ingramcontent.com/pod-product-compliance
Lightning Source LLC
Chambersburg PA
CBHW081152270326
41930CB00014B/3126